Atlas of ADVANCED ORTHODONTICS

Anthony D. Viazis, DDS, MS

In Private Practice, Plano (Dallas), Texas USA

Visiting Professor, University of São Paulo, Bauru, Brazil

Former Associate Professor, University of Southern California

Former Assistant Professor, Baylor College of Dentistry

University of Minnesota

Atlas of
ADVANCED ORTHODONTICS

A Guide to Clinical Efficiency

W.B. Saunders Company
A Division of Harcourt Brace & Company
Philadelphia London Toronto Montreal Sydney Tokyo

W.B. SAUNDERS COMPANY

A Division of Harcourt Brace & Company

The Curtis Center
Independence Square West
Philadelphia, Pennsylvania 19106

Library of Congress Cataloging in Publication Data

Viazis, Anthony D.
    Atlas of advanced orthodontics : a guide to clinical efficiency / Anthony D. Viazis.
        p.   cm.
    ISBN 0–7216–7637–5
    1. Orthodontics—Atlases.   I. Title.
RK521.V49   1998
617.6′43′00222—dc21   97–29321

ATLAS OF ADVANCED ORTHODONTICS   ISBN: 0–7216–7637–5

Printed in the United States of America

Last digit is the print number: 9   8   7   6   5   4   3   2   1

To the memory of my brother,
Panos

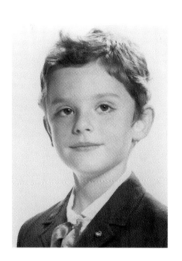

Preface

*A*tlas of Advanced Orthodontics: A Guide to Clinical Efficiency presents a colorful step-by-step approach to diagnose and treat orthodontic cases specifically and efficiently. By applying diagnostic and treatment procedures that are clear; predictable; and based on the latest research of diagnosis, cephalometrics, and clinical application, the clinician and student of orthodontics are certain of providing patients with the latest knowledge of orthodontics. *It is a guide to what works and works well.*

This book is a great addition to the best-selling *Atlas of Orthodontics*, as it takes the reader a step further. While *Atlas of Orthodontics* familiarizes one with the state-of-the-art generalities in modern orthodontics, *Atlas of Advanced Orthodontics: A Guide to Clinical Efficiency* focuses on direct patient care through a system of therapy and treatment techniques that improve clinical efficiency and maximize the effectiveness of patient care. The clinician learns how to utilize light, biological forces through the new superelastic wires and the new triangular brackets to reduce patient discomfort, shorten treatment time, and minimize the potential risk of iatrogenic root resorption.

This book, the first of its kind on efficiency of orthodontic therapy, emphasizes ways to treat cases with new material technology by using systems and techniques that reduce variation, combine the initial phases of treatment, provide plenty of time to finish cases, and make the overall practice of orthodontics fun and exciting.

Anthony D. Viazis, DDS, MS

Acknowledgments

I wish to thank the following individuals and institutions:

From the USA

The University of Southern California, Department of Orthodontics, Dr. Glenn Sameshima, DDS, PhD, Assistant Professor (for his contributions to video cephalometrics and figures 17–34); all the graduate students who worked very hard on the clinical cases that I supervised; and Dr. Peter Sinclair, DDS, MS, Professor and Chairman for his wise suggestions; from Dallas, Texas, Drs. Lorin Berland (for his contributions of figures 555–566) and Elizabeth Jaynes (for her contributions of figures 575–578); and Dr. Michael LaFerla of Joplin, Missouri (for his contributions to Friction research and figures 136–140).

From Europe

The University of Santiago in Compostella, Spain (for contributing figures 131, 132, 135); the University of Thessaloniki, Greece; the University of Münster, Germany; the University of Geneva, Switzerland; and the University of Kuopio, Finland, along with the orthodontic societies of Sweden, Finland, Greece, Italy, Spain, Holland, and Belgium for their interest in the new technology.

My brother, Dr. Angelo D. Viazis from Athens, Greece, for his excellent review of the literature and his assistance in the preparation of the chapters on Retention Facts, Cosmetic Dentistry, Functional Appliances, and Oral Hygiene.

Dr. M. Dalili, from the University of Kuopio, Finland, for his excellent PhD thesis on orthodontic discomfort.

From South America

The University of São Paulo, Bauru Dental School, Brazil, Dr. Guilherme RP Janson MSc, PhD, MRCDC, Assistant Professor; Décio Rodrigues Martins MSc,

PhD, Full Professor; José Fernando Castanha Henriques MSc, PhD, Associate Professor; Marcos Roberto de Freitas MSc, PhD, Associate Professor; Amaldo Pinzan MSc, PhD, Associate Professor; Renato Rodrigues de Almeida MSc, PhD, Assistant Professor (for their excellent clinical work and contribution of figures 82–85, 248–308, 528–552, and the chapter on functional occlusion and occlusal adjustment).

Dr. Luiz Carlos de Mesquita Cabral (for contributing figures 86, 309–322, and 487–517) and Dr. Evelyn Alvez of Santos, Brazil and the Orthodontic Society of the Dominican Republic.

Dr. Maiara L. Hister of Porto Alegre, Brazil for her assistance in the preparation of the chapters on Root Resorption and Cosmetic Dentistry.

I would also like to thank my office staff for all their hard work with all of our patients, and Tracy A. Pace, for her assistance in word processing and compilation.

Contributors

Chapter 4

Glenn T. Sameshima, DDS, PhD
Assistant Professor
Department of Orthodontics
University of Southern California
Los Angeles, California

Chapter 14

Michael R. LaFerla, DDS, MS
Private Practice
Joplin, Missouri

Chapter 17

Renato Rodrigues de Almeida, MSc, PhD
Assistant Professor
Bauru Dental School
University of São Paulo
Bauru, Brazil

Marcos Roberto de Freitas, MSc, PhD
Associate Professor
Bauru Dental School
University of São Paulo
Bauru, Brazil

José Fernando Castanha Henriques, MSc, PhD
Associate Professor
Bauru Dental School
University of São Paulo
Bauru, Brazil

Guilherme RP Janson, MSc, PhD, MRCDC
Assistant Professor
Bauru Dental School
University of São Paulo
Bauru, Brazil

Décio Rodrigues Martins, MSc, PhD
Full Professor
Bauru Dental School
University of São Paulo
Bauru, Brazil

Almado Pinzan, MSc, PhD
Associate Professor
Bauru Dental School
University of São Paulo
Bauru, Brazil

Contributors

Biography

*D*octor **Anthony D. Viazis** holds his dental degrees from the University of Athens and Baylor College of Dentistry. He received his specialty training in orthodontics and Master of Science from the University of Minnesota where he was awarded "Teacher of the Year" after his first year of teaching. He served on the faculty at Baylor College of Dentistry for four years. He received his title of Associate Professor from the University of Southern California. He is a Visiting Professor at the University of São Paulo, Bauru, Brazil. He maintains a full-time private practice of orthodontics in Dallas (Plano), Texas. He has published numerous clinical and research articles in the *American Journal of Orthodontics* and *Dentofacial Orthopedics*, the *Journal of Clinical Orthodontics*, and other dental publications. He lectures nationally and internationally. He is the author of the best-selling book *Atlas of Orthodontics: Principles and Clinical Applications*, by W.B. Saunders, and the inventor of the Triangular Bioefficient Bracket System (Viazis System) distributed by OrthoSystems, Inc. (OSI). Dr. Viazis' triangular braces have been featured on national television on *CBS This Morning* and over 80 news stations around the country. He is a member of the American Association of Orthodontists, the American Dental Association, the International Association for Dental Research, the Dallas County Dental Society, Who's Who Worldwide and Who's Who of American Inventors.

> *The future of orthodontics in the arena of increased technological advances is indeed very bright.*
>
> ANTHONY D. VIAZIS

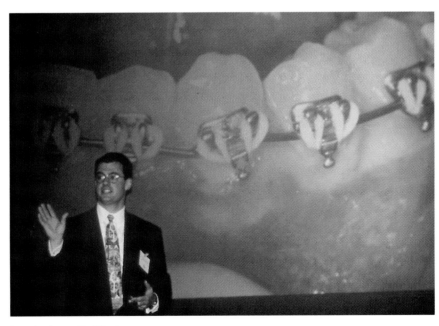

Dr. Anthony D. Viazis

Contents

Introduction

*E*fficiency in the everyday clinical practice of orthodontics is an absolute requirement for success in the contemporary environment of patient service. Efficiency leads to continuous room for practice growth through increased productivity. The utilization of the most modern methods and materials allows the clinician to serve more patients in the same time frame. Decreased variation and greater automation lead to increased productivity and thus to improvement of both quality and quantity of patient care through the reduction of chairside time and treatment duration.

In dealing with the human body, which is a biological mechanism, we always try to use the lightest forces possible to minimize iatrogenic root resorption. The new wire–bracket technology allows us to reduce the forces we use to move teeth and thus achieve a more biological intervention in less time and with less patient discomfort.

The overall objective of the diagnosis and treatment described in this book is a shorter initial treatment phase for an increase in the time available to finish and individualize the final outcome. It is an end-user (patient) friendly system as well as a user-friendly (doctor) approach with simple and efficient mechanotherapy. With the new orthodontic materials, we now have the capability to get through the initial time-consuming phases of orthodontic mechanotherapy that burn out both patient and clinician, and get to the exciting finishing stages of therapy with ease and comfort (individualizing therapy). As the treatment becomes easier and more convenient the patient is excited because he or she sees the beautiful changes of his or her smile early on in therapy and, thus, becomes very cooperative.

As this book is one of the first to present the new technology in orthodontics, one must keep in mind the words of Machiavelli: "There is nothing more difficult to take in hand, more perilous to conduct, or more uncertain in its success, than to take the lead in the introduction of a new order of things." One must also remember the words of Schopenhauer: "All truth goes through 3 steps: first, it is ridiculed, second it is violently opposed and finally, it is accepted as self-evident." As clinicians, scientists, and doctors we all share a common responsibility: the well-being and health of the public. This is why we should always evaluate new therapies with an open mind. As long as they have been shown to work clinically and have passed the test of independent university research, we should welcome them with open arms. As Plato said, "We can easily forgive a child who is afraid of the dark; the real tragedy in life is when men are afraid of the light."

Efficient orthodontic mechanotherapy means quality of patient care. As contemporary orthodontics enters a new era of individualized treatment with reduction in variation and enhancement of system effectiveness and productivity, the future of orthodontics in the arena of increased technological advances is, indeed, very bright. The constant change in this age of information and knowledge through critical clinical observation and research data will bring the art and science of orthodontics to horizons never before imagined.

For educational seminars or other information you may communicate directly to:

2317 Coit Road, #D
Plano, Texas 75075
tel: (972) 867-9473
fax: (972) 985-8481
email: topwire@orthosystems.net
website: www.orthosystems.com

Anthony D. Viazis, DDS, MS

Diagnosis

I

Clinical Evaluation

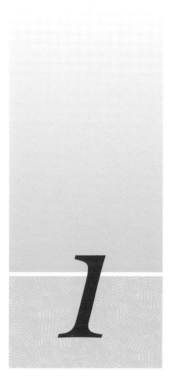

*T*he diagnosis of any efficient orthodontic treatment starts with the patient's chief complaint (Figure 1). The immediate question in the clinician's mind should be whether the patient's chief complaint may be addressed while at the same time obtaining a Class-I canine relation (Figure 2). It is a Class-I cuspid relation that is the cornerstone of a properly finished orthodontic case (Figure 3). The final molar relation may be Class-I, II, or III. Thus, the following decisions will have to be made: nonextraction versus extracting treatment for adolescent patients, the possibility of orthognathic surgery, especially for adults, and the indication for expansion and growth modification for patients in the mixed dentition.

In contemporary clinical orthodontics, patients appreciate a full smile, with teeth showing from corner to corner of the lips, and full vertical exposure of the incisor crowns along with 1 to 2 mm of soft tissue showing above those teeth (Figure 2). The profile is preferred a little fuller than in years past, with the lips on or slightly in front of a line connecting the middle of the nose with the chin (Figure 4). Extractions ought to be avoided if possible if the patient has thin lips.

The dental clinical evaluation should follow, where general notes, an evaluation of the intraoral soft tissue, teeth, and oral function, and a panoramic radiograph are made. Any operative, periodontal, and endodontic work (if needed) should be completed before initiation of orthodontic treatment, whereas any temporomandibular joint (TMJ) pain or dysfunction should be addressed before the onset of orthodontic treatment.

The chief complaint must have been met by the end of treatment or the patient will not be happy, even if the orthodontic therapy is of the highest standards. If the patient or guardian has unrealistic expectations that may not be met with treatment, the clinician ought to educate him or her so that he or she understands the limitations of the various therapeutic modalities in modern orthodontics.

In a study on the changes in the molar relation between the deciduous and permanent dentitions, it was concluded that 61.6%, 34.3%, and 4.1% of patients end up with a Class-I, Class-II, and Class-III permanent molar relation, respectively (Figures 5–8). The (overbite) OB and the OJ (overjet) in the incisor area should be approximately 2 mm.

A clinical way to assess crowding is by "eyeballing" it, taking into consideration the average width of the various teeth (bicuspids, 7 mm; canines, 8 mm; lower incisors, 5–6 mm; upper centrals, 10 mm; upper laterals, 7 mm). By subtracting how much tooth material is blocked out of the arch or is in a crowded position, one may very quickly evaluate the space that is needed to obtain good tooth alignment. This is undoubtedly a very crude method, but one that clinical experience has shown to approximate (± 1 mm) to the exact discrepancy.

Single-tooth crossbites are usually dental in nature. Multiple-tooth crossbites are anterior or posterior and usually skeletal in nature. Anterior tooth crossbites may be "pseudo Class-III" (due to a shift) or "true Class-III" (true skeletal). Posterior crossbites are unilateral or bilateral. Most multiple-tooth crossbites are bilateral and are due to a constricted maxilla. Multiple-tooth crossbites should be corrected as soon as possible to avoid the possible development of a skeletal malocclusion or abnormal eruption of teeth, as well as to improve the patient's esthetics.

A large percentage of patients have mesial-distal tooth size discrepancies, approximately 13.8% and 9.2% for the mandibular and maxillary dentitions, respectively. Such discrepancies, if left untreated, could lead to future posttreatment relapse, especially in the mandibular incisor area. Interproximal reduction will, in most cases, alleviate such discrepancies toward the end of treatment.

If the tooth size discrepancy is in the posterior teeth, then they may be selectively reduced in width, enough to obtain a Class-I cuspid relation. Interproximal reduction should be done in the upper or lower arch to make these teeth fit in relation to their counterparts, toward the last stages of treatment.

If a compromise must be made because of the patient's malocclusion (to achieve a Class-I relation), it may be best to leave the lower midline off by 1 to 2 mm (a lot of patients do not show their lower teeth on smiling). The upper dental midline should coincide with the facial midline for an esthetically pleasing smile.

A thorough functional evaluation is an essential part of the development of the patient's stomatognathic problem list. Habits should be evaluated carefully; their duration and intensity may be more important than the actual presence of an abnormal condition. Although the literature is replete with statements that airway impairment alters facial and dental growth, there is substantial evidence to the contrary. What may be an excellent therapeutic modality for one patient does not indicate that it will have the same effect in most patients. Although there seems to be a weak tendency among mouth breathers toward a Class-II skeletal pattern, increased anterior facial height, high mandibular plane angles, and retroclined incisors—all characteristics of a long face—a more thorough analysis of respiratory pattern is required to support the decision for clinical intervention. A referral to the patient's physician or ear, nose, and throat specialist may be appropriate.

The most superoanterior position of the condyle is musculoskeletally the most stable position of the joint (centric relation). The position of the mandible where the relation of opposing teeth provides for maximum occlusal intercuspation is called *centric occlusion*. This, ideally, should coincide with centric relation; this is what the clinician should strive for during orthodontic treatment. In most cases, a slight discrepancy of about 1 mm also can be acceptable, where the position of the mandible in centric relation is slightly behind its position in centric occlusion.

One should keep in mind that as much as 50%, if not more, of the population has one sign of joint dysfunction (e.g., noise, tenderness, etc.); the female-to-male ratio ranges from 3:1 to 9:1, and only 5% of the patients with signs and symptoms are in need of TMJ therapy. During the TMJ examination of the patient, the clinician should look for possible sore muscles (in the neck and mouth area) and any "clicking" noises (with the use of a stethoscope or digital palpation), as well as any deviation on opening and closing (the mandible deviates toward the side of an anteriorly dislocated disk), any signs of bruxism and clenching (it is nighttime clenching that in many cases results in morning headaches), and the overall strain-level status of the patient.

If temporomandibular dysfunction (TMD) symptoms arise during orthodontic treatment, observation and common sense are the best approaches. If the symptoms are painful, it may be necessary to modify active therapy: reduce forces, stop headgear, eliminate direct mandibular distalizing forces, minimize interarch elastic use, and eliminate gross occlusal interferences, preferably by bite plates that open the bite by 1 or 2 mm, and occlusal coverage splints. These measures allow sore muscles and joints to recover so treatment may proceed.

The role of orthodontic treatment in either precipation or prevention of TMD remains questionable. Orthodontic treatment does not appear to pose an increased risk for development of TMJ sounds or symptoms, regardless of whether extraction or nonextraction treatment strategies are used. The original growth pattern that caused the teeth to be selected for extraction—rather than the extraction itself—is the most likely factor responsible for the frequency of TMD reported years later. Bicuspid extractions and subsequent orthodontic treatment do not lead to irreparable damage of TMJ muscles. Condylar position is unrelated to extraction treatment and to bite depth. It has been shown that the claim that bicuspid extraction and incisor retraction of necessity lead to unsightly profiles and distal mandibular displacement cannot be supported. People who have undergone orthodontic treatment have a significantly lower clinical dysfunction index than those who have not. Orthodontically treated patients are not more likely to develop TMD signs while undergoing treatment. A relation between either the onset of TMJ pain and dysfunction and the course of orthodontic treatment or the change in TMJ pain and dysfunction and the course of orthodontic treatment has not been established.

Figures 1, 2

This patient's chief complaint was her narrow smile. This complaint was successfully addressed after 14 months of orthodontic therapy.

Figure 1

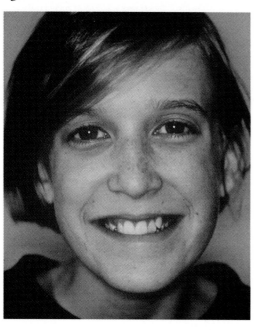

Figure 2

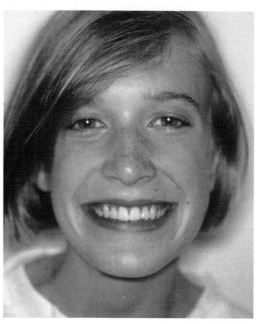

Figure 3

A Class-I canine relation in which the upper canine occludes in the embrasure between the lower first premolar and lower canine. Contemporary orthodontic mechanotherapy leads to treatment results that are based on the six keys to normal occlusion: (1) a Class-I molar relationship (or Class-II or III, as long as the canine is in Class-I); (2) crown angulation (tip)—the gingival portion of the crown of the teeth is distal to the incisal portion in most individuals; (3) crown inclination (torque)—anterior crowns have an anterior inclination, whereas posterior crowns have a lingual inclination; (4) absence of rotations; (5) absence of spaces; and (6) the plane of occlusion should be flat or have a slight curve of Spee. The first objective of orthodontic mechanotherapy in the anteroposterior dimension is the attainment of a Class-I canine relationship. This not only results in a stable, functional occlusion, but it ensures a good overbite and overjet relationship when no tooth size discrepancy is present. The upper central and lateral incisor roots should be slightly convergent, and the remaining upper teeth should show a distal inclination, except for the second molars, which should be mesially tilted. The lower incisors should be upright, and the other lower teeth should be increasingly distally inclined as one moves posteriorly.

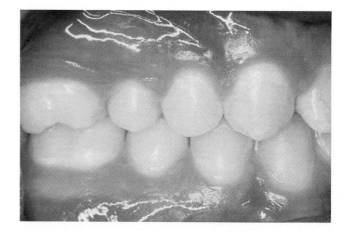

Figure 4

The contemporary profile with slightly full, procumbent lips.

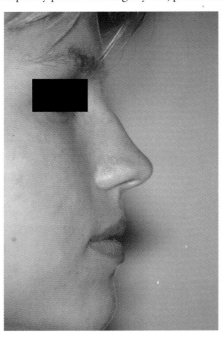

Figure 5

A Class-I molar relation (upper molar slightly behind lower).

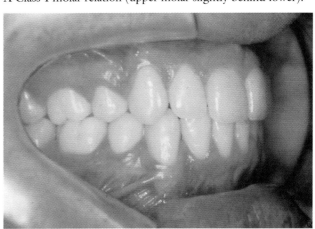

Figure 6

A Class-I molar relation results in a normal overbite/overjet relation of 2 mm.

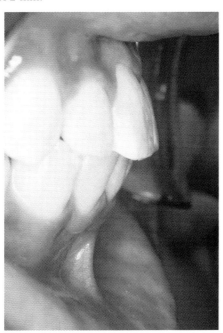

Figure 7

A Class-II molar relation (upper molar in front of Class-I position) results in excess overbite/overjet relation.

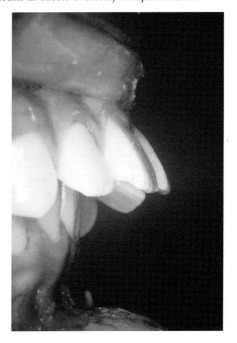

Figure 8

A Class-III molar relation results in an inadequate overbite/overjet relation.

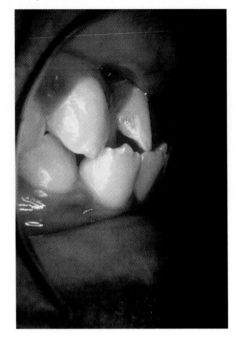

Cephalometrics

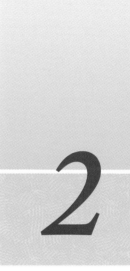

*F*acial examination is the key to diagnosis. Orthodontic complications nearly always stem from errors in diagnosis, not from failures in execution of treatment. After the preliminary dental clinical information is obtained, the evaluation continues with the examination of the face from the frontal and profile views. The patient is instructed to sit upright and look straight ahead into the horizon or directly into a mirror on the wall. This position, called the *natural head position* (NHP), is the position in which the patient carries himself or herself in everyday life. Therefore, this is the reference position we should use in our examination. In this position the pupils of the eyes are centered in the middle of the eyes, defining the line of vision or *true horizontal* (TH). The TH line should be parallel to the floor (Figure 9).

   Natural head position has been established over the past 30 years as the most appropriate reference position for cephalometric radiography. No difference was found between the variability of the Frankfurt horizontal and the sella–nasion line with regard to the horizontal plane. The large variation of both intracranial reference lives, related to NHP, confirms their relative unsuitability as cephalometric references for clinical purposes. Findings indicate that a horizontal line, related to natural head position, adjusted to natural head orientation when indicated, presents the most reliable basis for cephalometric analysis. It has been shown that it is related to the correct natural body posture and alignment with the cervical column, is based on the line of vision, and is determined by the overall head and body balance when the individual looks straight ahead. The reproducibility of NHP has been shown to be within the clinically acceptable spectrum of variance of 4°, which is certainly much better than the 26° variability of the Frankfurt horizontal and sella–nasion plane among different individuals.

   An NHP radiograph is taken with the patient in the cephalometer looking straight ahead into a mirror. The patient is observed from the side to ensure that the pupil is in the middle of the eye (Figure 9). In the event that the patient states that he or she is in NHP but the pupils are not centered in the middle of the eyes, the clinician should correct the head position. Any habitual tendency for an individual to keep the head in an "unnatural" flexed or extended position must be observed, and it may be necessary to "correct" the registered head position. Recently, using tracings of facial profiles, observers made independent, subjective estimations of NHP in 28 adults. The results of these estimations were compared with recordings of NHP obtained through photographic registration of the same subjects. Only minor average differences (between 0° and 1.4°) were found between the two methods. Estimation of NHP may, therefore, be performed with acceptable accuracy in most cases. Head posture needs to be standardized during cephalometry. Thus, it is the clinician, and not the patient, who determines the final position, and therefore this final position may be called the standard treatment position (STP).

The ear rods should be placed directly in front of the tragus so that they lightly contact the skin, establishing bilateral head support in the transverse plane. Lateral cephalostats with ear rods alter the position of the head and neck during postural recordings. Subjects extend their heads and necks higher with ear rods in place than they do without ear rods. The patient should be comfortable and relaxed, and the head should not be tilted or tipped. The correct position is confirmed by checking the patient from the front. The nose piece is then placed so that it lightly contacts the skin, to establish support in the vertical plane. The three light contact points secure the patient in NHP. After a final check, the radiograph is taken. The entire procedure should take only 1 to 3 minutes. The determination of an esthetic true horizontal by visual inspection of the patient's face has been shown to be highly reproducible and to have more relevance to the soft tissue than does the Frankfurt horizontal.

The following are some cephalometric landmarks used in this clinical cephalometric analysis (Figure 10):

A-point (A): An arbitrary point at the innermost curvature from the anterior nasal spine at the crest of the maxillary alveolar process.

Anterior nasal spine (ANS): The process of the maxilla that forms the most anterior projection of the floor of the nasal cavity.

B-point (B): An arbitrary point on the anterior profile curvature from the mandibular landmark, pogonion, to the crest of the alveolar process.

Gnathion (Gn): The most downward and forward point on the profile curvature of the symphysis of the mandible.

Gonion (Go): The most posterior and inferior point on the angle of the mandible that is formed by the junction of the ramus and the body of the mandible.

Labialis inforioris (LI): An arbitrary point at the vermilion of the lower lip.

Labialis superioris (LS): An arbitrary point at the vermilion of the upper lip.

Menton (Me): The most inferior point on the symphysis of the mandible.

Middle of the nose (No): The midpoint between the subnasale and pronasale on the true horizontal, projected on the inferior outline of the nose.

Nasion (N or Na): The most anterior point of the frontal suture.

Pogonion (P or Pg): The most anterior point on the symphysis of the mandible.

Posterior nasal spine (PNS): The process formed by the most posterior projection of the juncture of the palatine bones in the midline.

Pronasale (Pr): The tip of the nose.

Sella (S): A constructed point in the middle of the sella turcica.

Soft tissue menton (Me'): The point on the lower contour of the chin opposite to the hard tissue menton.

Soft tissue pogonion (P'): The most anterior soft tissue point of the chin.

Stomion (St'): A point at the interlabial junction of the mouth where the upper and lower lips connect.

Subnasale (Sn): The point at which the base of the nose meets the upper lip.

V-point: The midpoint of the distance between A-point and Sn.

The significance of soft tissue evaluation lies in the importance of the role that dentofacial attractiveness plays in our society. As clinicians, we need to make sure that we do not compromise the soft tissue for a good occlusion, and vice versa. A soft tissue evaluation from the facial and profile view is essential to have a comprehensive understanding of the patient's esthetic characteristics (Figure 10).

More significance should be attached to soft tissue profile evaluation than to cephalometric analysis in orthodontic diagnosis and treatment planning. A parallel to the true vertical from No and the line NoPg' define the *V-angle* (Figure 11). This angle denotes the convexity of the face. The mean ± SD is –13° ± 4°. The NoPg' line (Steiner's S-line)—the line connecting the middle of the nose (No) and the chin (Pg)—should barely touch the upper and lower lips. Steiner's S-line has been used for more than 25 years as a quick reference of the anteroposterior position of the lips relative to the nose and chin.

The V-angle is similar to the facial contour angle (FCA), but provides a better indication of profile convexity because it concentrates on the lower half of the face and takes into account the size of the nose. It does not allow the size of the nose to affect the evaluation of lip position as much as the E-line (the line connecting the tip of the nose to the chin, PrPg') does, because it uses only half of the nose length.

A perpendicular to the TH through V-point (*V perpendicular*) should pass through the soft tissue pogonion. The distances between the two perpendiculars to the TH from the V- and Sn-points provide the posterior and anterior limits of the harmonious soft tissue chin position range (Figure 10).

The assessment of the relative anteroposterior position of the maxilla and the mandible is done with the true horizontal Wits (Figure 10). If points A and B are projected on the TH through perpendicular lines, points A and B are defined, respectively. The AB distance is defined as the *true horizontal Wits* versus the original *Wits on the occlusal plane*. The TH Wits provides a more clear relation of the anteroposterior position of the jaws relative to each other than does the original Wits, which can sometimes be affected by the inclination of the occlusal plane or by the inclinations of the Frankfurt horizontal. The mean ± SD for this measurement is 4 ± 2 mm.

It has been shown that there is no measurement or set of measurements that can be used successfully to predict growth rotation (vertical jaw position), even by experienced clinicians. The mandibular plane angle (GoMe-TH) is one of the most widely used cephalometric measurements. This angle may sometimes mask the true growth tendencies of the mandible because of extensive remodeling changes occurring at the angle of the mandible and the symphysis. High values indicate a backward growth rotator, and low ones indicate a horizontal growth pattern. The mean ± SD is 24° ± 4°. The angle decreases approximately 2° ± 2° from childhood to adulthood (Figure 10).

Another useful measurement is the maxillomandibular plane angle. This measurement highlights the divergence or conveyance of the two jaws as they grow. The mean ± SD is 28° ± 4° (Figure 10).

The inclination of the functional occlusal plane is demonstrated with the occlusal plane angle (Figure 10). The angle between TH and the functional occlusal plane (OP) is derived from the lower molar and bicuspid cusp tips and locates the teeth in occlusion relative to the rest of the face. As with the mandibular plane, high values indicate a backward and low values a forward growth rotation. The mean ± SD is 8° ± 2°.

The inclination of the upper incisor (UI) to the maxillary plane is shown with the UI angle. This is the angle formed from the long axis of the UI and the ANS/PNS line. The mean ± SD is 110° ± 5°.

The inclination of the lower incisor (LI) to the mandibular plane is obtained with the LI angle. The long axis of the LI and the GoGn plane form this angle. The mean ± SD is 92° ± 5° (GoMe can be used as well).

In the case of suspected facial asymmetry, a posteroanterior cephalometric film is evaluated (Figure 12). A tracing is made and vertical planes are used to illustrate transverse asymmetries. Lines are drawn through the angles of the mandible and the outer borders of the maxillary tuberosity. Vertical asymmetry can be observed readily by drawing transverse occlusal planes (molar to molar) at various vertical levels and observing their vertical orientation. If a significant skeletal asymmetry is detected, orthognathic surgery may be incorporated in the treatment plan. A more thorough evaluation would then be needed by the oral and maxillofacial surgeon.

A computerized cephalometric analysis is now available (Figures 13, 14). This makes the evaluation and overall analysis very efficient.

Figures 9, 10

The natural head position (NHP) or standard treatment position (STP). The angle formed from the cranial base to the true vertical (perpendicular to the true horizontal or line of vision) with the T (tubercullumn sella)–Na (nasion) line may be used in future radiographs to orient the patient. The remaining measurements comprise a very practical assessment of the teeth to the profile. These cephalometric reference lines and measurements comprise the original Viazis cephalometric analysis (VCA). The line through the "V" point is used simply as a reference to assess chin position and evaluate possible genioplasty for cosmetic purposes. This book does not focus on orthognathic surgery. If a patient is a candidate for such surgery, then a more thorough analysis may be used (see Viazis AD: *Atlas of Orthodontics*. Philadelphia: WB Saunders, 1993).

Figure 9

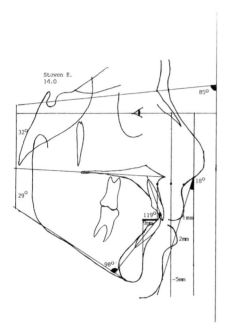

Figure 10

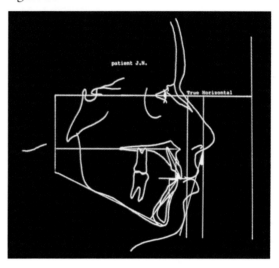

Figure 11

The most important cephalometric measurement, the esthetic V-angle. It quantifies the profile in the face.

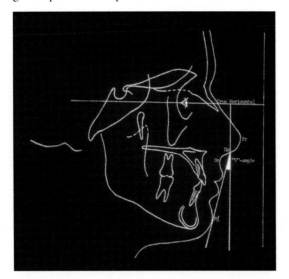

Figure 12

Visual analysis of a posteroanterior cephalometric film is performed easily with vertical lines through some key areas.

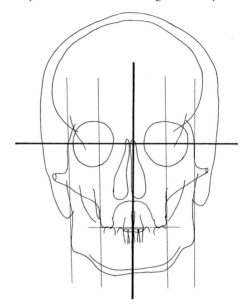

Figures 13, 14

A modification of the original VCA is available in the Orthotrak (OMS) Cephalometric Software (Norcross, GA). It mainly substitutes the incisor inclination measurements with assessment of tooth protrusion based on the nasion (NA, NB, NPg). This analysis also notes the upper incisor exposure for assessment of the vertical relation of the smile. This modified VCA places emphasis on the relation of the existing dentition to the soft tissue in the assumption that no orthognathic surgical procedure is to be done. Therefore, the clinician tries to maximize the positive relation of the dentition to the face.

Figure 13

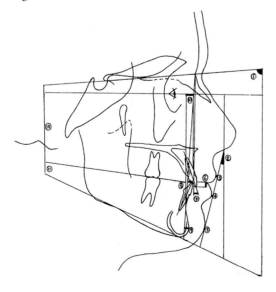

Figure 14

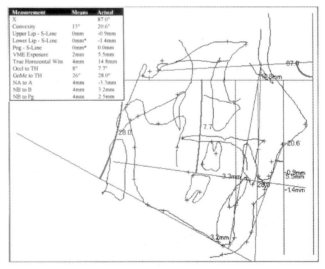

Measurement	Means	Actual
X		87.0°
Convexity	13°	20.6°
Upper Lip - S-Line	0mm	-0.9mm
Lower Lip - S-Line	0mm*	-1.4mm
Pog - S-Line	0mm*	0.0mm
VME Exposure	2mm	5.5mm
True Horozontal Wits	4mm	14.8mm
Occl to TH	8°	7.7°
GoMe to TH	26°	28.0°
NA to A	4mm	-3.3mm
NB to B	4mm	3.2mm
NB to Pg	4mm	2.5mm

Section I: *Diagnosis*

Growth Analysis

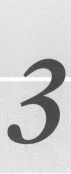

*I*t has been well documented that the anterior wall of the sella turcica and the cribriform plate remain unchanged after the fifth year of life. This means that no growth or remodeling changes affect these areas of the cranial base by the time the first permanent tooth erupts in the oral cavity, which is most likely the earliest time an orthodontic consultation or intervention may be needed. Growth changes of the facial skeleton can be carefully evaluated by superimposing cephalometric radiographs on these stable structures. Yet the various existing superimposition techniques do not concentrate on using this portion of the cranial substrate. All of the other areas currently used are subject to growth changes. Even the most popular superimposition technique—superimposition on the SN line by registering on S (sella)—expresses growth more anteriorly than it actually occurs. A reason for avoiding the use of the aforementioned stable areas has been the difficulty in accurate location of the cribriform plate and the small dimension of the anterior wall of the sella turcica.

The following superimposition approach offers a sound and practical way of incorporating these structures in the evaluation of facial growth. Three points are used to define the triangle (Figures 15, 16):

1. *T-point:* The most superior point of the anterior wall of the sella turcica at the junction with tuberculum sella. It can be quickly located on the radiograph and does not change with growth, as does the sella (S).
2. *C-point:* The most anterior point of the cribriform plate at the junction with the nasal bone. Even though the cribriform plate is not easily detectable, the C-point is quite clear on the cephalometric radiograph at the most posterior tip of the nasal bone. Na-point (nasion) may be used if the C-point is not easily detectable.
3. *L-point:* The most inferior (lower) point of the sella turcica. This point also defines the most posterior point of the anterior wall of the sella turcica.

The triangle incorporates in its area the whole anterior wall of the sella turcica and extends over a large area that includes all of the anterior and part of the middle cranial base. The three points selected are at the greatest distance from each other within stable structures. This provides the clinician with a large marking area. By registering on the T-point and superimposing on the anterior wall of the sella turcica and the stable TC line (cranial base line), a solid formation is provided through the shape of the triangle in both the anteroposterior and vertical planes for a practical and dependable evaluation of facial growth. The purpose of the triangle is to provide the clinician with a quick, solid, visual orientation of the most stable areas of the cranial base (Figure 16).

It is preferable to obtain a cephalometric radiograph of all growing patients at the age of 9 or 10 years or at the initial visit at the office. Just before orthodontic treatment is to begin and at least 6 months after the initial radiograph, a second cephalometric radiograph gives the clinician the ability to compare the two and evaluate facial growth. When superimposing the two triangles as described previously, the two lower sides of the triangles may not necessarily fit right on top of each other, especially because of the L-point (because of slight remodeling changes in the area). Focus should be placed, in the order of registering, on (1) the T-point, and superimposing on (2) the inner structure of the triangle (anterior wall of the sella turcica), and (3) the TC line. This recommended methodology simplifies the procedure of the "best-fit" approach while recognizing the limits of realistic expectations with a superimposition technique.

A line connecting the T-point with gnathion (Gn) is defined as the G-line, which may be used as a growth line. The advantage of the G-line over the other ones that use the sella is attributed to the stable position of the T-point versus the unstable S (sella point) because of growth and remodeling. In addition, the T-point is an anatomic landmark, whereas the sella is a constructed one (the middle of the sella turcica).

The mean ± SD of the angle formed between the G-line and the TH (D-angle) is $58° ± 4°$. Growth is downward and forward along this line (D-angle stable with growth). Backward rotation of the G-line (by registering at the T-point) with growth indicates vertical growth (D-angle increases). Anterior rotation of the G-line with growth indicates a forward horizontal growth pattern (D-angle decreases).

The angle between the TC line (stable cranial base line) and the *true vertical* (TV) may be established on the first tracing of a patient. Any additional radiographs of this patient taken to evaluate either growth changes or treatment effects may be oriented so that the *TC-TH angle* remains constant. In this way, the patient is treated to his or her initial NHP, established in the beginning of treatment, regardless of postural, behavioral, or surgical effects. In other words, the patient is treated to a constant NHP based solely on the line of vision, which is established when the pupil is in the middle of the eye and the individual is looking straight ahead.

In understanding the importance of craniofacial growth and its role in the development of malocclusion, one needs only to comprehend the role of dental compensation to the skeletal growth pattern.

Malocclusions stem from the inability of teeth to compensate for an abnormal skeletal pattern. If we were to look at several skeletal open-bite cases, we would notice that the anterior dentition (incisors) is retroclined (tipped lingually) and has supererupted in most of these cases. This is nature's attempt to compensate for the abnormal skeletal growth pattern that has created the open bite (backward rotation) with dental movement that decreases the extent of the open bite over the years. The opposite would take place in a deep-bite patient. The teeth would flare labially in an effort to decrease the deep overbite relations. Of course, this is not clearly visible in all cases, because other factors play a role in the overall appearance of the dentition (e.g., muscles, soft tissue, tongue–lip equilibrium, tongue function, parafunctional habits).

The aforementioned differences in nature's dental compensations involve the vertical plane. If we were to look at skeletal development problems in the anteroposterior dimension, we would notice a similar compensatory pattern. In a Class-III mandibular prognathism patient, as the negative overjet (underjet) develops, the upper incisors tip labially and the lower incisors tip lingually in an effort to keep as normal an overjet relation as possible. It is as if the teeth are trying to "hold on" while the mandible grows excessively anteriorly.

The diagnosis of such problems may become more complicated when we have abnormal skeletal development in both dimensions, vertically and anteroposteriorly, such as the Class-III, open-bite patient presented previously. A thorough cephalometric evaluation along with proper superimposition of serial radiographs help in locating the extent of the problem in both dimensions.

An example of dental compensation is given in the situation of two patients who may have the same skeletal open-bite tendency, but one has a normal open bite/overjet of 2 mm and the other an open bite. The teeth of the first patient compensated by supereruption of the anteriors, whereas they did not for the second patient. In the past, when orthognathic surgery had not yet developed to its current level, clinicians would correct such malocclusions by completing nature's work, that is, extrude the teeth (in the case of an open bite) to close the bite.

Another example of the role of dental compensations involves the decision of extraction versus nonextraction on two individuals who have the same crowding and dental appearance, but one has an open-bite tendency (backward rotation) and the other a deep bite (forward rotation). Nature tends to compensate in open-bite cases by supererupting the anterior teeth and tipping them lingually. Nature compensates for a deep bite by flaring the anteriors labially. We would rather extract teeth to resolve the crowding in an open-bite case, because this treatment modality would allow us to tip the rest of the teeth lingually (working along with nature's attempt to compensate) to close the bite. Extractions in a deep-bite case should be avoided, if possible, because the remaining teeth would move lingually and make the bite deeper. Therefore, nonextraction approaches should be investigated for deep-bite cases.

Finally, in evaluating the patient's growth, the clinician ought not ignore the nose. The growth of the nose has been the focus of many investigations over the past 30 years because of the important role that nasal development plays in orthodontic treatment planning. Class-I subjects tend to have straighter noses, Class-III subjects reveal a concave configuration of the nose along the dorsum, and Class-II individuals exhibit a more pronounced elevation of the nasal bridge (greater dorsal hump), leading to the increased convexity observed in the Class-II patient. Most investigators state that nasal growth for girls continues until the age of 16 years. In addition, very small increments of nasal growth have been reported between the ages of 18 to 22 years, and as late as 26 to 29 years of age. Developmentally, the greatest change occurs in the anteroposterior prominence of the nasal tip in both sexes, and because the forward positioning of the nose is greater than that of the soft tissue chin, it appears that the lips are receding within the facial profile. The patient ought to be informed of the potential effects of his or her nasal growth on the profile.

Figures 15, 16

The cranial base triangle, the growth axis, and directional angle. The eruption of the upper incisor should follow the growth axis in a parallel fashion.

Figure 15

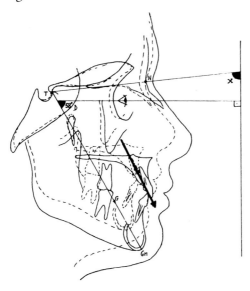

Figure 16

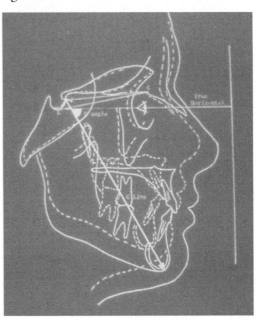

Video-Imaging

Glenn T. Sameshima

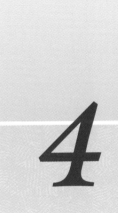

In an episode of the old television show, *Star Trek*, Captain Kirk's opponent is not a jingoistic alien biped, but a computer designed to replace him on the *Enterprise*. Naturally, Kirk prevails since the computer is unable to make a command decision requiring pure human judgment. In a sense, our practices are our starships, and we sit in the command chair. Technology often seems threatening and the revolution in computing has not left orthodontics alone. No successful practice today is without a desktop machine performing some time-saving repetitive task, whether it be simple word-processing or scheduling many appointments for several offices at once. However, computers have made less of an impact on the clinical aspects of our practices. The reason is clear—orthodontics is as much an art as a science, and the clinical decision-making process requires full use of Kirk's "human" ability in judgment. That said, however, computers are becoming an essential part of chairside clinical practice.

What exactly is video-imaging? Video-imaging is simply the process of capturing an image and storing it in the computer for future use. The term "video" as used here has a dual meaning: (1) the typical video signal from a camcorder or television set and (2) video in reference to the way the computer handles graphics internally.

How is video-imaging used in clinical practice? Video-imaging has two primary uses in orthodontics. First, video-imaging is one of the most formidable tools the clinician can use in patient communication and education. Second, video-imaging is an important adjunct in diagnosis and treatment planning. An additional use of video-imaging is the archiving, or storage, of records in the mythical paperless office.

How hard is video-imaging to learn? Like most computer programs, there is a bit of a learning curve involved; however, there is no prerequisite that the doctor or staff be computer geniuses. Unless someone in the office is a computer hobbyist, it is best to regard these systems as simply another sophisticated piece of office equipment, that is, something that you don't tinker with unless there is a problem. (It is often the case that a little knowledge is more dangerous than none, and the folks who have developed these wonderful programs will tell you that the untrained computer "expert" fouls up more systems than anyone else!)

The better companies will train you and your staff (patiently!), and have toll-free technical support available during business hours. A yearly contract for support and upgrades must be maintained with the company and is well worth the cost.

Good video-imaging systems need a good computer system. Usually, the computer and related items ("hardware") are "bundled" with the computer program ("software") that tells the computer what to do. Essential components include a fast computer, a color monitor with a large viewing area (17 inches or larger), a color printer, a color video camera, and an input device such as a scanner or digitizer. There are several good systems on the market and all share some common features. A separate room or large area should be dedicated to the imaging system. The office should anticipate the need to upgrade or change the hardware in 3 to 5 years. Why? The quality of the pictures, both the one you see on the screen and the one printed on paper will improve greatly during that time period. Improvements are often added as upgrades, and periodically a completely new version comes out that requires new hardware to use the new features. Everyone has a fascination with computer hardware; perhaps it is because we become so gadget-oriented in dental school. However, it must be emphasized that the prime consideration in a good system is not the hardware, but the software and the support that comes with it. Avoid the advice of your colleagues who are unable to talk about computers without lapsing into heavy use of jargon and technospeak!

The most useful feature of the video image is in communication. Most patients seeking orthodontics and orthognathic surgery cite facial esthetics as the number-one reason. Studies have shown that patients have a much better idea of what to expect from the surgery, and, in fact, that the actual outcome is usually better than the predicted one. Patient satisfaction is also reported to be higher with imaging than with line drawings.

The accuracy of the surgical predictions has been studied and it has been shown that the programs are more accurate in the horizontal direction than the vertical; however, nearly all measurements in the systems tested were accurate to within 1 mm. This is well within the range of what would be considered clinically accurate. Figure 17 shows a composite of the presurgical initial profile (left), the predicted profile (middle), and the actual postsurgical profile (right) from a recent study.

The uses of video-imaging with orthognathic cases are almost limitless. The clinician can view the projected outcome of several different options—single jaw, double jaw, chin (genioplasty), and so forth. Imaging also allows both the practitioner and the patient to see the whole face—plastic procedures such as rhinoplasty, malar augmentation, and removal of excess skin and tissue under the chin can be simulated using the image-altering tools in the programs. (Considerable training and experience are necessary for the clinician to be able to make these forecasts with confidence and accuracy.) Figures 18 and 19 show the initial and predicted views of the patient's profile in anticipation of an orthognathic surgical procedure (mandibular advancement). Figures 20 and 21 demonstrate the anticipated changes in a Class-III mandibular prognathic surgical case. The patient can readily see the changes in jaw profile and can participate in the surgical decision-making process. Figure 22 illustrates the use of the "compare" feature of the program just as it appears on the computer. The patient can see the presurgical view (left), a predicted single-jaw (middle), and a predicted double-jaw alternative (right). As the patient views the image, the doctor explains the advantages and disadvantages of each procedure. During the discussion, the doctor uses the images to point out specific areas that will be most affected by the choice of surgery. Active participation in this phase of treatment is crucial to good patient–doctor communication and avoiding later misunderstandings.

Figure 23 is a frontal view of a patient who presents with a chief complaint of gummy smile and underbite. The diagnosis confirms vertical maxillary excess, horizontal maxillary deficiency, and true mandibular prognathism. Figure 24 shows the image altered with simple cut-and-paste tools to show the patient what might be expected from an osteotomy procedure to address the vertical excess. Ideally, the doctor and surgeon who work together on these cases should have the same type of imaging system in their respective offices to facilitate communication with each other. It is possible to transmit these images and patient information over the telephone lines if the computers have the necessary hardware (a modem) and software installed.

Figure 25 is a typical patient with the primary complaint of crooked teeth. Using the "smile library" feature of the imaging program, the operator quickly outlines the smile with the mouse, clicks on a menu choice, moves the smile outline to the "library" of smiles, clicks on the appropriate one (for size, shape, and color), and "pastes" it back into the patient (Figure 26). Hard copy of the new smile can be generated and given to the patient—with a disclaimer, of course! These images can also be easily pasted into a premade form letter, which comes with the program, that can be printed out and sent to the referring dentist or the patient with the clinical findings and treatment plan. The smile library also contains smiles with metal and clear appliances on the teeth. If a patient wants to know what his or her teeth will look like with appliances on, it is very easy to paste one of these smiles in place and show them the look. Not all of the images saved in the computer have to be standard orthodontic views. For example, one can save an image documenting poor hygiene. It takes a little more work, but you can put this picture in the poor-hygiene letter you send to the patient's parents.

Another interesting and useful feature is the "growth forecasting" routine. Predicting growth is usually an imprecise exercise to begin with, but the clinician can make good use of these programs in helping patients understand treatment goals. A Class-II patient who is about to begin her adolescent growth spurt is shown in Figure 27. Parents often wonder what is meant by language such as "growth modification," "restraint of maxillary growth," "redirecting condylar growth," and the like. Figure 28 shows the forecast growth (assuming no treatment) for a 3-year time period. (The computer uses sophisticated mathematical algorithms based on a built-in database of averages to "grow" the face.) The large screen makes it easy for the parents and patient to see the increasing overjet and poor profile that will result if no intervention takes place. Conversely, growth forecasting can also be used in those patients who grow poorly—typically a patient with a good profile in Class-I occlusion who grows into a Class-III—to show what growth should have taken place and did not, thus causing extended treatment time and changes in treatment plans. As our understanding of the growth process improves with scientific investigation, the value of these forecasting features will increase substantially.

We now discuss how these pictures are put into the computer. There are several ways to accomplish this. Most of the systems were designed with live video capture in mind. In live video capture, the patient is seated with the head in natural rest position and a camcorder is used to view the profile on the computer. When the operator is satisfied that the head and lips are positioned properly, a key is pressed and the image is captured (i.e., saved in the computer). The operator can look at the saved image immediately, and if something is not right, he or she can recapture at once. Frontal views of the patient are captured next. Intraoral views of the dentition may also be captured using a camcorder, but most prefer to use photography. In some offices, even though this may be the patient's first visit, the clinician will use the smile library as discussed previously to help with the initial consultation. We would like to believe that the patient hears and understands everything we say during the initial visit, but a picture truly is worth a thousand words.

Many offices still prefer to send their patients to an x-ray laboratory for the radiographs and photos. To bring these into the computer, one of several alternatives must be picked and somebody in the office must be trained in the chosen method. The methods for entering cephalometric information and photographs are different. Color photographs are usually input by putting the camcorder on a special mounting device or "copy stand." A little trial and error, and a standard height for the camcorder is established with proper lighting (color-balanced). Each photo is then placed under the camcorder, and when it looks right on the screen, it is captured just as in live-video capture. The disadvantage here is in the quality of the picture; the live capture nearly always looks better.

An alternative to using the camcorder is to scan the picture in. This is becoming a more acceptable way to put the images in and the newer versions of the imaging systems are beginning to incorporate this method. A scanner is a device that works in a way similar to a copy machine. There are scanners that are designed just for family photos and produce good image quality; this will probably soon be an option for image capture.

Still another method for the photographs is the use of a digital camera. These cameras look like real cameras, but instead of film, they capture the picture onto a small computer chip. Digital photography is a nascent but potentially dominant field, and this will eventually be the way all nonradiographic images are taken.

Many clinicians prefer to take 35-mm color transparencies (slides). These are easily input using a slide video device (really a camcorder built specifically to look at slides) or a slide scanner.

Radiographs, specifically, lateral cephalometric radiographs, can be saved, but usually the goal is input of the landmarks and structures so that cephalometric analyses can be run. The popular systems have three ways of getting this data. (1) The ceph is captured with a camcorder or, better, a black and white video camera dedicated to this purpose; (2) the ceph is scanned using a flatbed scanner (see previous discussion); and (3) the ceph is placed on a "digitizer" and the landmarks and structures are identified and entered directly (Figures 29, 30). For methods 1 and 2, the landmarks and structures are identified on the computer screen and traced using the mouse and keyboard. Research has shown that method 3 is the most accurate; however, one system has a way to enhance the ceph image on the screen to improve identification of difficult areas.

Video-cephalometry, as aptly termed by Sarver (1996), is the standard in cephalometrics. The consistency and sheer speed of computing the analyses instead of doing the measurements by hand has made the latter as obsolete as banding anterior teeth. The clinician can pick from a number of different analyses, or he or she can make a customized one. Hard copy can be produced on a color printer (Figure 31). If a treatment prediction is desired, the next step is to precisely overlay the tracing onto the patient's image (Figure 32). Then, using the treatment planning feature, the clinician selects a movement of the teeth or jaws and the computer morphs the soft tissue to the forecast position. The amount of surgical movement is calculated by the system in millimeters. Angular movements, such as uprighting of teeth, are recorded in degrees. These measurements are an invaluable aid in the treatment planning process, but rely on good records and skillful and exact placement of the tracing on the image.

There are many other excellent, useful features in these systems. Superimposition of tracings from different times (or different patients) is easily accomplished with your choice of reference structures (Figures 33, 34). Libraries of different tracings can be catalogued and saved. Patient letters incorporating images can be quickly produced without going into a separate word-processing or publishing program. Some systems allow models to be input and saved; occlusal views of the models can be analyzed for crowding and tooth size discrepancy. For the clinician who prefers not to image the patient in-house, a few x-ray laboratories have become imaging centers where all of the pictures and images are collected, the cephs digitized, and the information sent to the clinician on computer disk or transmitted via modem.

Although these systems should be reserved specifically for video-imaging, some of the companies have added other functions outside of video-imaging. The interactive CD-ROM is invaluable in patient education, and several companies have made excellent ones for orthodontics. Patients can be led through a discussion of subjects specific to their treatment, such as functional appliances, palatal expansions, headgear wear, and so forth. These CD-ROMs are particularly good because they incorporate pictures, sound, and animations—thus getting the full attention of the TV generation. Professional journals and other educational materials designed for the clinical practice are becoming increasingly available on CD-ROM, and simplify the search for information of interest. A single CD-ROM, for example, can easily hold 10 years of journal articles, including tables, graphs, and photographs.

In summary, the use of computers in our practices will continue to improve the way we run our offices and treat our patients. Discussion of hardware and current features is difficult because of the incredible speed of change in the industry. The key is to focus on how this technology can help us simplify and improve our daily lives, and, most important, how this technology can benefit our patients.

Figure 17

Presurgical, video-imaging predicted, and postsurgical profiles of a patient. (Courtesy of Dr. Glenn Sameshima.)

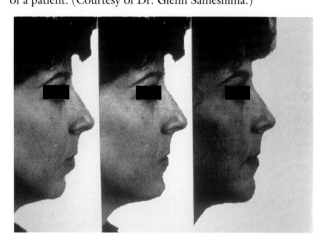

Figures 18, 19

Initial profile of a patient and the predicted posttreatment profile of the patient through video cephalometrics. (Courtesy of Dr. Glenn Sameshima.)

Figure 18

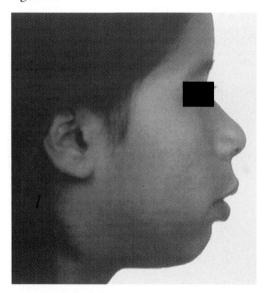

Figure 19

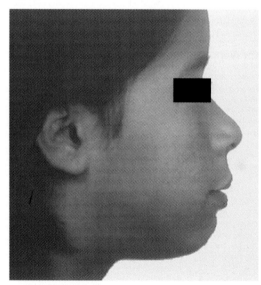

Figures 20, 21

Anticipated changes in a Class-III patient. (Courtesy of Dr. Glenn Sameshima.)

Figure 20

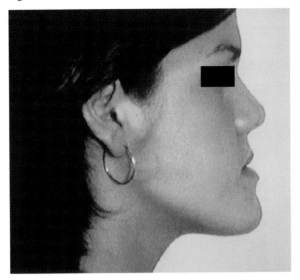

Figure 21

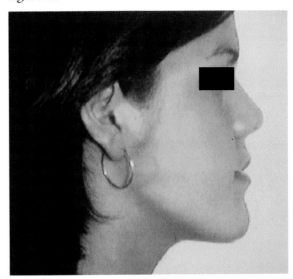

Figure 22

As the patient views his or her images on the computer screen, the doctor explains the advantages and disadvantages of each procedure. (Courtesy of Dr. Glenn Sameshima.)

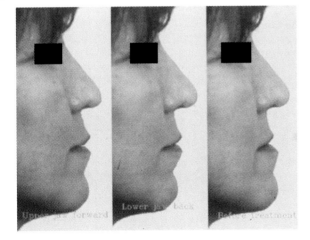

Anticipated changes in a patient with a gummy smile and underbite. (Courtesy of Dr. Glenn Sameshima.)

Figure 23

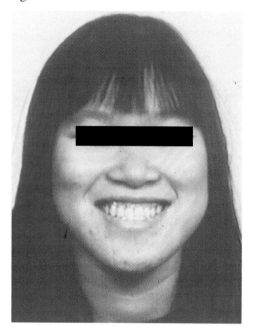

Figure 24

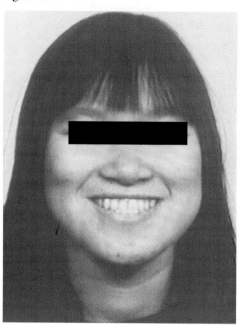

Figures 25, 26

"Cut-and-paste" smiles from the "smile library." (Courtesy of Dr. Glenn Sameshima.)

Figure 25

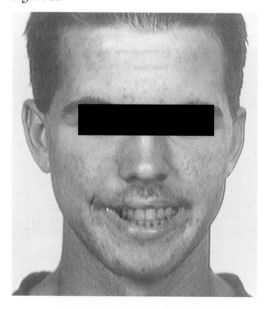

Figure 26

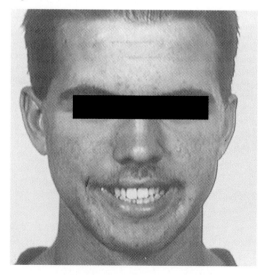

Figures 27, 28

Anticipated changes in a Class-II patient. (Courtesy of Dr. Glenn Sameshima.)

Figure 27

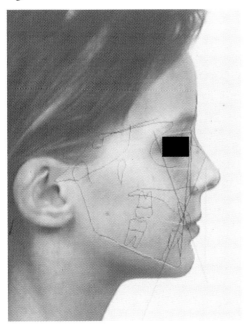

Figure 28

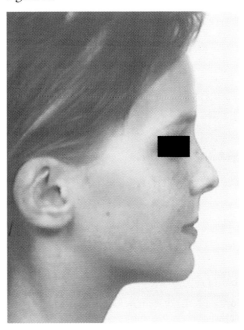

Figures 29, 30

Computer entry of cephalometric data. (Courtesy of Dr. Glenn Sameshima.)

Figure 29

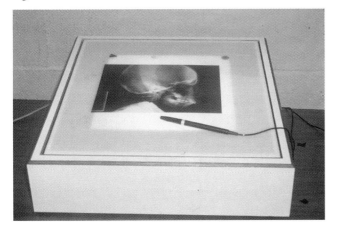

Figure 30

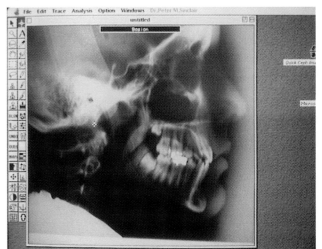

Figure 31

Color printer. (Courtesy of Dr. Glenn Sameshima.)

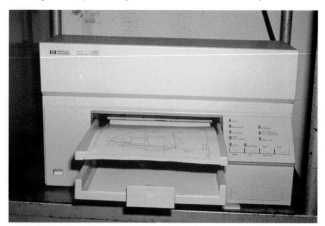

Figure 32

Overlay of tracing onto the patient's image. (Courtesy of Dr. Glenn Sameshima.)

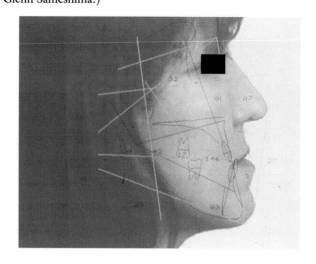

Figures 33, 34

Superimpositions to determine treatment or growth changes. (Courtesy of Dr. Glenn Sameshima.)

Figure 33

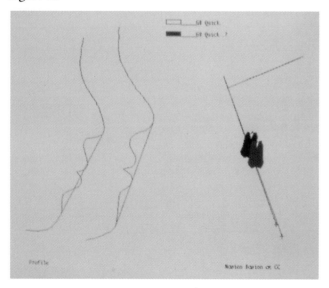

Figure 34

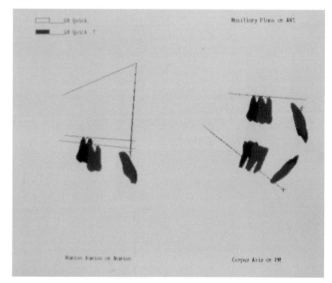

Treatment Planning

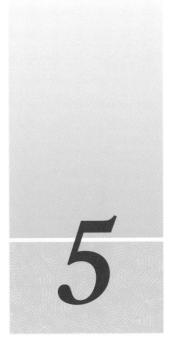

The primary objective in orthodontics is the attainment of a Class-I cuspid relation after treatment, when the upper cuspid occludes in the embrasure between the lower first bicuspid and cuspid. With this goal in mind, the following general treatment patterns may be applied in orthodontics.

Class-I: Most patients with Class-I cases who seek orthodontic therapy have minor, moderate, or severe crowding, accompanied by various intra-arch discrepancies that are easily corrected orthodontically. Minor and moderately crowded cases are usually resolved with the tooth recontouring (TR) technique. When we have a Class-I extraction case (severe crowding, impacted teeth, bimaxillary protrusion, dental open bite or open-bite tendency cases), the objective is the presence of the Class-I cuspid and molar relation. If there is severe crowding in both arches, extraction of all first premolars will alleviate the problem and the Class-I cuspid and molar relation can be maintained. If there is severe crowding on the upper or lower arch only, then the first premolars in both arches may need to be extracted to preserve a Class-I cuspid relation.

Class-II: Class-II cases are either division 1 (flared upper incisor, excess overjet) or division 2 (retroclined upper central incisors, labially displaced laterals, and no overjet). By uprighting the retroclined upper central incisors in a division 2 case, we turn it into a division 1 case. Therefore, the treatment approach for both is similar. The treatment strategy with such cases depends on the patient's age. In mixed dentition, nonextraction mechanotherapy that would move the upper posterior teeth distally is the treatment of choice. In the adolescent permanent dentition, some clinicians may try to do the same as in the mixed dentition, whereas others would extract the upper first premolars and finish a Class-II molar and Class-I cuspid relation. In the adult patient, the ideal treatment in most cases would be nonextraction and uprighting of the central incisors, followed by a mandibular advancement orthognathic surgical procedure that would improve facial esthetics. (Class-II patients usually have a retrognathic mandible.) If the patient refuses surgery, the treatment of choice would be extraction of the upper first premolars.

Class-III: In a recent investigation of 302 adult Class-III individuals, it was reported that almost one third of the sample had a combination of maxillary retrusion and mandibular protrusion. Maxillary skeletal retrusion with a normally positioned mandible is found in 19.5% to 25% of Class-II patients. Mandibular protrusion, commonly cited as the major skeletal aberration in individuals with Class-III malocclusion, was found in only 18.7% of the total sample.

In another study, a combination of maxillary retrusion and mandibular protrusion was found in 22.2% of the sample. Forty-one percent of this entire sample (59 of 144) also had long lower face height. Clearly, even in children and adolescents, a Class-III malocclusion does not indicate some typical facial skeletal pattern. Rather, it can be the result of any of several combinations of aberrations in the craniofacial complex. There is a tendency toward a morphologic difference between the mandibles of Class-III and Class-I individuals. This difference occurs early. The increase in vertical lower anterior facial growth occurs later and is not typically present in early childhood. In young patients (5–11 years of age) with maxillary deficiency, the treatment of choice is protraction facemask therapy. In patients with mandibular prognathism, it is best to wait until completion of growth for a mandibular setback orthognathic procedure. This eliminates the possibility of a second surgery because of late or excessive growth of the mandible in the late teens or early twenties, especially in boys. In the event that any dental problem exists, orthodontic therapy alone may be undertaken (depending on the case), followed by retainers.

If the crowding is in both arches, extraction of all premolars would lead to a Class-I cuspid and molar relation. If it is in the upper arch only, extractions of the upper first premolars would alleviate the crowding but worsen the Class-III situation, because the anterior teeth would have to be retracted further posteriorly. Thus, the options available to us are (1) maxillary advancement or mandibular setback surgery to obtain a Class-I cuspid relation, or (2) lower first bicuspid extractions to end up with a Class-I occlusion.

The preceding situation is exactly the opposite, in terms of extraction patterns, to the Class-II lower severe crowded case. If the crowding is in the lower arch only, extraction of the lower first premolars will result in a Class-I cuspid and a Class-III molar relation.

The assessment of the patient's condition results in one of the following:

1. Do nothing;
2. Treat by nonextraction;
3. Treat by extraction;
4. Consider orthognathic surgery if indicated; or
5. Consider expansion/growth modification if needed.

Furthermore, any one of the preceding options is based primarily on whether a Class-I canine relation can be achieved. Therefore, one of the following will be considered:

1. If nonextraction therapy is chosen, one must secure the canine in Class-I relation as the teeth are brought into position. The crowding (if any) will be resolved with a combination of tooth recontouring or tooth alignment with fixed appliances or expansion. The objective is a broad smile from corner to corner (Figures 35–41).

2. If the crowding is severe, especially in open-bite tendency cases, then extraction of premolars is considered. If we have a Class-I canine relation, then four premolars are usually extracted. If we have a Class-II canine relation, then only two upper premolars need be removed to bring the canines into a Class-I relation. Lower incisor extraction or recontouring of the lower dentition will help alleviate any lower crowding. If we have a Class-III canine relation, then only two lower premolars need be removed. Upper expansion or recontouring will help alleviate any upper crowding.

3. Orthognathic surgery may be indicated in a few cases as long as the desired result is significantly more pleasing to the patient over a nonsurgical treatment modality. This book focuses on contemporary orthodontic therapy that does not involve surgery.

4. Upper and lower expansion of the arches along with biteplate or headgear therapy may be used in the mixed dentition (Figures 42, 43) for arch width gain or growth modification in an attempt to treat the patient with nonextraction and possibly nonsurgically later on.

Suture Expansion

Figures 35, 36

Maxillary expansion involves the separation of the two halves of the upper jaw as the mid-palatal suture widens. Contemporary maxillary expansion appliance with bands on the first molars and extended anterior wires to the premolars. By turning the screw once a day for a month, the arch's widened. The separation of the suture is evident from the midline diastema between the central incisors.

Figure 35

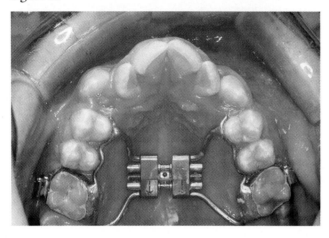

Figure 36

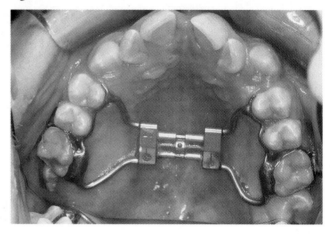

Figure 37

The screw is sealed and the expansion is held for 2 to 3 months. After that, fixed appliances are placed to align the teeth.

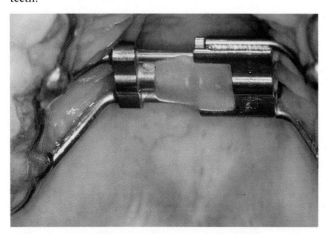

Figures 38, 39

Narrow upper arch resulting in a narrow smile.

Figure 38

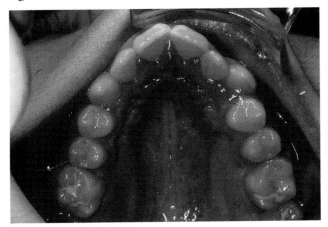

Figure 39

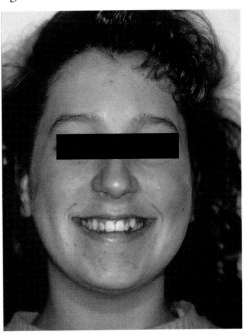

Figures 40, 41

Same patient after arch expansion. Note the broad smile from corner to corner.

Figure 40

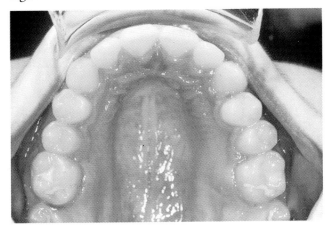

Figure 41

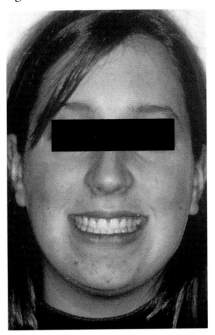

Figure 42

Lower arch expansion is best accomplished in the mixed dentition, before the full eruption of the lower permanent canines. In this way, the alveolar bone is expanded as the canines erupt and position it further buccally.

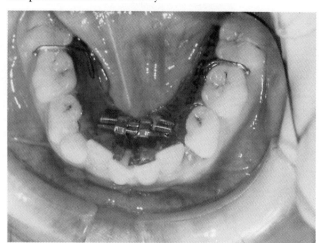

Figure 43

The screw is expanded once a week for 6 to 7 months.

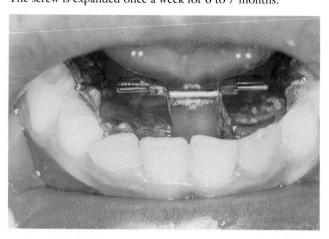

Efficient Treatment Timing

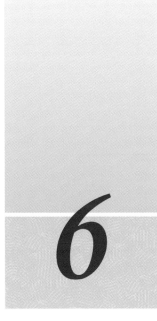

*T*he ideal time to treat a malocclusion has been often debated in the orthodontic literature. One of the dilemmas facing the orthodontic clinician is whether to intervene before the eruption of the permanent dentition. It has been well documented that some malocclusions, such as skeletal crossbites (resulting in a functional shift) are best treated as early as possible; others, such as Class-II malocclusions, are best left untreated until a later stage of dental transition to best use growth and avoid patient burnout, overtreatment, an excessive number of appointments, and overall inefficient therapy.

One may approach the treatment of malocclusions based on the concept of "efficient treatment timing" (Table 1). According to this concept, a malocclusion should be treated as soon as possible when postponement of treatment would lead to severe functional or esthetic concerns. On the other hand, certain malocclusions may be treated at a later stage as long as any later treatment would have the same effects as early treatments but involve less overall treatment time. Thus, the therapeutic benefits are maximized with optimal doctor time, continuous patient cooperation, and patient satisfaction.

Habit control, functional crossbite correction, and alleviation of possible crowding, especially in deep-bite cases, should be initiated as soon as they are detected. A deficient maxilla (Class-III) should be protracted (facemask) as soon as the upper permanent first molars erupt, and often right after the eruption of the upper permanent incisors. True mandibular prognathism is best treated surgically after completion of growth. Mild mandibular prognathism can be effectively addressed in the deciduous dentition with chincap therapy. Open- and deep-bite tendencies should be addressed by the late mixed dentition stage. The author agrees with Gianelli (1996) that Class-II malocclusions, especially those requiring distal molar movement, may be best treated by nonextraction with continuous treatment of 1.5 to 2 years that starts in the late mixed dentition, especially on the eruption of the upper first premolars. Finally, any limited treatment (single-tooth crossbite, diastema, spacing) can be addressed individually per patient at any age. Any dysfunction or pain to the TMJ should be addressed as soon as it is detected. Fixed-appliance therapy should use the new superelastics, wires, springs, and efficient bracket designs.

Table 1. Treatment Time Table

Problem	Efficient Treatment Period			
	Deciduous Dentition (4–6 yr)	Early Mixed (6–8 yr)	Late Mixed (8–11 yr)	Permanent (Growing)
Habit	Discontinuation			
Crossbite with shift		Maxillary expansion (sutural)		
Crowding		E-space control Expansion		Fixed appliances
Class-II			Headgear/springs (alveolar) Functional	Fixed appliances
Class-III maxillary deficiency	Facemask			Fixed appliances
Class-III mandibular prognathiom	Chincup			Fixed appliances
Deep bite		Space maintenance/biteplate		Fixed appliances
Open bite (skeletal)			Headgear/vertical Corrector tooth guidance	Fixed appliances
Limited treatment		Any time		
Temporomandibular joint dysfunction treatment		Conservative approach on detection		

In conclusion, the objectives of any treatment before eruption of all permanent teeth are to correct the skeletal discrepancy between the jaws and improve function and facial esthetics by allowing them to develop normally, to create an ideal overbite and overjet relation, to align the anterior permanent teeth (incisors) and reduce the chance of trauma to these teeth, to improve the width of the dental arches, and to reduce the risk for (1) extraction of permanent teeth on normal eruption of the full permanent dentition, and (2) surgery (in severe cases). Unattended orthodontic problems can lead to impairments in speech and chewing and loss of or trauma to teeth. Orthodontics can enhance a person's self-esteem as treatment brings teeth, jaws, and soft tissue into correct position. This is accomplished with the good level of cooperation that a child demonstrates during this period.

A treatment will be successful only when the patient and guardian are satisfied with the result of therapy. This is always accomplished in the environment of caring that our young patients need. Every effort should be made to minimize the level of discomfort at any phase during treatment and maximize the esthetic changes due to therapy.

Root Resorption: A Review

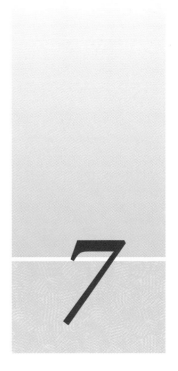

*I*n conventional orthodontic mechanotherapy, apical root resorption is a common idiopathic problem. The treatment duration and mechanical factors definitely influence root resorption. The magnitude of the orthodontic force is believed to be an important factor, not only for the magnitude of the tooth movement but for any tissue damage. It is believed that too strong a force will cause increased damage to the roots. Friction may be a significant influence on the amount of applied force required to move a tooth in the mouth. Hence, archwire and bracket selection may be an important consideration when posterior anchorage is critical. (This consideration is discussed in greater detail in Chapter 10, Figures 78–85.)

Most studies report that the severity of root resorption is directly related to treatment duration. *Treatment time should be as short as possible.* Rudolph (1940) reported that 40%, 70%, 80%, and 100% of the patients in treatment demonstrated some root resorption after 1, 2, 3, and 7 years of active treatment, respectively. No severe resorption was detected at the end of treatment in teeth without resorption after 6 to 9 months.

Some reports claim that not only the magnitude but the duration of the applied force is an aggravating factor for root resorption. The duration of force has even been regarded as a more critical factor than the magnitude of the force, especially in connection with long treatment periods. Increased length of treatment time, considered by itself, was positively associated with increased root resorption ($p = 0.013$). This finding is consistent with the findings of most of the earlier studies. According to Brezniak and Wasserstein (1993a and b), of 16 earlier studies examining this relation, 13 found that resorption increased as a function of treatment time, whereas the remaining three found no such association.

Independent university studies in Europe and the United States show that the new triangular design demonstrates up to 10 times less frictional force compared with conventional brackets, regardless of the wire being tested. In most cases this means reduced risk of potential iatrogenic root resorption (due to less force/treatment time), in addition to greater *comfort* during tooth movement. According to Schwartz (1932), *when pressure decreases below the optimal force (20–26 g/cm²) root resorption ceases.* Based on the latest research (see chapter on

Friction), the new triangular brackets (Bioefficient) and superelastic wires (Bioforce) provide such low forces.

Rosenberg (1972) reported that teeth with incompletely formed roots showed less root resorption than those with completely formed roots. Teeth with incomplete root formation at onset of orthodontic treatment showed root lengthening during active treatment, yet did not reach their "normal" tooth length. Treated and untreated random samples showed no correlation between gender and root resorption. According to studies, females are more susceptible to root resorption. The idiopathic female-to-male root resorption ratio was 3.7:1. An appliance–gender interaction was evident for some teeth, with the edgewise male group showing more root resorption than the "low-friction" male group ($p < 0.05$). Individual variation in biologic response to orthodontic forces may in part explain variation, and genetic predisposition may be another important predisposing factor. The side effect of treatment may be due to individual variation, and not to "round tipping." Apical root material loss was greater in treated females (0.73 mm) compared with treated males. Dougherty (1968a and b) speculated that this may reflect the difference in root maturity because the male is chronologically less mature than the female, and the male roots are less susceptible to the traumatic effects of orthodontic stress. Hormonal differences were not advocated by researchers who found an existing disparity between male and female.

One study reports that the incidence of root resorption increased from 4% before orthodontic treatment to 77% after conventional treatment. Another related study showed increased root resorption to bone architecture resulting from hormonal and nutritional imbalance during growth. Yet another study found no correlation between root resorption and malocclusion classification. Most studies report that maxillary teeth are more sensitive than mandibular teeth. The maxillary incisors are the teeth most affected by root resorption. The extent of movement in these teeth is usually greater than in others because of malocclusion, function, and esthetics. Their root structure and relation to bone and periodontal membrane tend to transfer the forces mainly to the apex. The most frequently affected teeth, according to severity, are the maxillary laterals, maxillary centrals, mandibular incisors, distal roots of mandibular first molars, mandibular second premolars, and maxillary second premolars.

There was no difference found in the extent of root resorption in patients treated with or without extractions. Higher stress causes more root resorption. According to Schwartz (1932), applied force exceeding the optimal level of 20 to 26 g/cm^2 causes periodontal ischemia, which can lead to root resorption.

The chances for root resorption of a lateral incisor adjacent to an impacted canine are significantly higher ($p < 0.001$) when the lateral incisor is normally sized. One could speculate that in these cases, the normal-sized and early-developing lateral incisor root obstructs the deviated eruption path of the canine, and consequently stands a considerably greater chance of being damaged by resorption.

The use of elastic forces may increase the risk of apical root resorption only on the tooth that supports the elastics, probably because of jiggling movements of the anchor teeth. Therefore it seems that biomechanically complex orthodontic treatment may lead to an increased risk for apical root resorption; use of elastics may be a risk factor for the teeth that support the elastics. The amount of root movement and presence of long, narrow, and deviated roots increase the risk for apical root resorption.

Root resorption at the microscopic level occurs in every patient who undergoes orthodontic treatment. In most cases, it is a mere blunting of the root apices. In some patients, it is more severe for reasons that seem to be idiopathic, with the exception of previously traumatized teeth, which are more susceptible to resorption and loss of vitality. Around 16.5% of patients have approximately 1 mm of resorption of the maxillary incisor teeth. Maxillary incisors have been reported to be the most susceptible to this severe resorption, with other teeth less affected. A recent study showed that 3% of patients have severe resorption (greater than one fourth of the root length) of both maxillary central incisors.

Less resorption is observed in patients treated before age 11 years, perhaps because of a preventive effect of the thick layer of predentin on young, undeveloped roots.

The longer the active treatment time, the greater the chance of severe resorption. Obviously, a patient with small, rounded roots is not a good candidate for excessive tooth movement. Iatrogenic root resorption is caused by jiggling teeth over long periods of time, indecisive treatment that causes changes in the direction of tooth movement, and proximating of the cortical plate. Class-III patients are overrepresented in the group with severe resorption. No relation has been found between the amount of root shortening and degree of intrusion achieved. Contact of maxillary incisors with the lingual cortical plate may predispose to resorption. In general, *treatment time is the most significant factor for occurrence of root shortening*. In a recent long-term evaluation of root resorption occurring during orthodontic treatment, it was shown that there are no apparent changes after appliance removal except remodeling of rough and sharp edges.

Impacted canines may cause resorption of the adjacent incisor teeth; thus, their extraction or uncovering and movement into the dental arch is necessary. Potential incisor resorption cases from impacted canines are those in which the cuspid cusp in periapical and panoramic films is positioned medially to the midline of the lateral incisor (0.71%). The risk of resorption also increases with a more mesial horizontal path or eruption.

Based on all the aforementioned research findings, it becomes clinically obvious that, by starting three-dimensional tooth movement with the new superelastic rectangular or square wires (Bioforce) that deliver different forces to different teeth (light in the front, heavier in the back) in the almost zero-friction triangular brackets (Bioefficient), jiggling movements and excessive forces are avoided, and thus the potential risk of root resorption is reduced. As the transition to the finishing stainless steel wire is made earlier in treatment, overall treatment time is shortened, and therefore it appears that the potential risk for root resorption is reduced.

A recent investigation undertaken by Janson et al. (1997) compares the apical root resorption after orthodontic treatment and the treatment time with standard edgewise, straight wire, and the Bioefficient (triangular) system. Pretreatment and posttreatment periapical radiographs of 90 patients (30 treated with the standard edgewise bracket, 30 with the straight wire, and 30 with the bioefficient system were studied). The long cone paralleling technique was used for all the posttreatment radiographs. The pretreatment radiographs were only used to standardize the sample, excluding those teeth that presented previous endodontic treatment or root resorption. The posttreatment radiographs were evaluated by the score method of Levander and Malmgreen. The non-parametric Kruskal-Wallis test was used to compare the amount of root resorption, and the analysis of variance was used to compare the treatment time among the three groups.

The Scheffé test was used for individual comparisons of the treatment time among the three groups. The Bioefficient system presented statistically significant less root resorption at the end of treatment. The standard edgewise system presented a longer treatment time than the straight wire and the bioefficient systems which presented similar treatment time. Treatment time with the bioefficient system was smaller than with the straight wire system, although not statistically significant.

In a study from Finland, Daili et al. (1997, PhD thesis), found that the faster tooth movement was also more comfortable. The study group consisted of 59 (42 female and 17 male, mean age 26.5 years, SD 10.7) patients at the beginning of their active orthodontic treatment at the dental clinic, University of Kuopio. The design of this study was approved by the Ethics Committee of the Medical Faculty of the University of Kuopio, Finland. The quality, severity, and duration of pain symptoms of patients subsequent to the placement of orthodontic separators and fixed appliances were assessed by a questionnaire. The methods that were developed for dentin hypersensitivity tests were adopted for evaluation of tooth response to orthodontic forces. Electrical pain thresholds were measured with a constant current electrical stimulator in μA. For the sensitivity tests an electrothermal device with cold probe was constructed in the technical center of the University of Kuopio. Alginate impressions for dental hard stone casts were taken at the beginning of the treatment and three months after the initial archwire placement; tooth movement was then measured using the Irregularity index (R. Little). In addition, panoramic and lateral cephalographs were taken just before the treatment and six months after placement of fixed appliances, for detection and evaluation of the type of tooth movement (tipping or bodily) and root resorption.

The results showed significant statistical difference in tooth movement between the two systems, giving the leading edge to the triangular bracket therapy system making it faster than the conventional system. The average space closure in extraction cases was found to be 2.8 mm at the third month when using the triangular bracket system.

On the third day after activation of initial archwire, the pain/discomfort reports in mastication of food and fitting of back teeth together were less statistically significant in the Bioefficient therapy triangular bracket system compared to the conventional system. The results indicate that using the triangular bracket system causes less pain and discomfort than conventional therapy as the orthodontic treatment progresses.

Functional Appliances

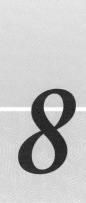

Growth modification is theoretically expressed in the following three ways: (1) by an increase or decrease in the size of the jaws; (2) by redirection, even if the absolute size remains the same; and (3) by acceleration of growth. Although histologically evident and statistically significant, an absolute change in size is clinically insignificant. Redirecting growth in another direction has been shown to be of some value. A patient with a severely prognathic mandible might benefit from redirection of his or her growth in a more downward than forward manner. Acceleration of growth shortens treatment time and provides a better jaw relation sooner. Correcting a skeletal problem through growth modification should begin 1 to 3 years before the adolescent growth spurt, so that the maximum effect may be obtained in the shortest possible time frame. This is done by use of functional and extraoral appliances.

The term "functional appliance" refers to a variety of removable appliances designed to alter the arrangement of the various muscle groups that influence the function and position of the mandible in order to increase its length. A number of clinicians believe that this is best achieved by 2- to 3-mm incremental advancements of the mandible every 4 to 5 months, because this decreases the risk of muscular fatigue as each new forward position of the mandible results in renewed growth stimulation of the condyle.

In general, the use of functional appliances remains controversial. Minimal bone growth increase (2 mm), along with the creation of dual bites in patients, puts them in an unfavorable position in the armamentarium of the modem practitioner.

Most functional appliances induce mandibular function in a predetermined position, usually 3 to 8 mm anteriorly to the centric relation position (Class-II correction). This stretches the soft tissue and muscles, which in turn transmit the resulting forces to the teeth (dentoalveolar changes) and to the skeletal substrate. Functional appliances may retard maxillary growth in the same modality as headgear. In addition, it has been shown histologically that new bone is formed in the posterior aspect of the glenoid fossa, which usually resorbs after the stimulus (anterior repositioning of mandible) is taken away.

The correlation between condylar growth and lateral pterygoid muscle activity was a constant finding in animal studies. It was proven that increased activity of this muscle was correlated with increased condylar growth. However, it might be the tension in the posterior part of the condylar capsule—caused by the activity of the lateral pterygoid muscle—that is responsible for increased condylar growth. The resultant tension of structures in the posterior part of the capsule decreased after a maximum level of activity 6 to 8 weeks after the start of treatment. A constant reactivation may, therefore, be important in obtaining a maximum condylar growth response.

Tipping of teeth and dentoalveolar changes are the effects of functional appliances. Class-II correction is the result of nearly 50% skeletal and 50% dental changes. Functional appliances that promote a Class-II dentoalveolar correction are the Activator, the Bionator, the Fränkel, the Twin Block, the Herbst, and the Jasper Jumper. The last two are fixed (nonremovable) appliances. Appliances that help to correct a Class-III problem use lip and buccal shield pads to relieve the maxillary dentoalveolar complex from any extreme pressure, so that it may grow to its full potential (Fränkel III). Such appliances require extreme patient cooperation to have any effect. A number of studies have shown that the average increase in mandibular growth was 2 mm. At the end of treatment with functional appliances, one might achieve a mean growth modification of 2 mm, which is clinically insignificant (6 mm of bone growth is necessary to correct a full Class-II malocclusion into a Class-I).

The best controlled clinical studies of functional appliance therapy have been unable to show clinically useful increases in mandibular length. Recently, it has been shown that bone formation at a histologic level does take place in the glenoid fossa after functional appliance therapy. The increased fibrous tissue of the disk posterior to the condyle appears to stabilize the anterior condylar displacement. This fibrous overgrowth (in conjunction with possible muscle splinting) may explain why the mandible cannot be manipulated back after functional appliance therapy, thus giving the false impression of a Class-II correction. Within a matter of months, such fibrous tissue resorbs and the mandible partially returns to its original position.

The dramatic results shown in some European studies required more than 2 years of full-time appliance wear. Other studies have demonstrated the effects of a headgear–functional appliance combination with similar results: improvement of the occlusal discrepancies, but necessitating great patient cooperation and the use of fixed appliances to finish the cases ideally. If this type of therapy is to be attempted, then the growth potential in the early mixed dentition would be as favorable or even better than in the pubertal age groups.

The full correction of Class-II, division 2 malocclusions into Class-I through the use of the Bionator functional appliance has been demonstrated in the literature, but, again, after very lengthy treatments of as much as 7 years (8–15 years of age) with 15 to 18 hours of wear a day. Arch expansion gained with the Fränkel appliance through the action of the vestibular shields (which displace the attachment of the lips and cheeks at the sulci in an outward direction, thus allowing the development of the apical base) seems to be more stable than the expansion seen with fixed appliance treatment. Again, the major disadvantage of the Fränkel therapy is the length of full-time wear (2.5–4 years) of a bulky appliance to obtain this desired result.

In a recent study on the changes in mandibular length before, during, and after successful orthopedic correction of Class-II malocclusions using a functional appliance, it was found that there was no significant difference after 4 years between the control and treated individuals. In addition, it was concluded that the greater the result, the greater the relapse potential. The main causes of relapse after Herbst treatment were a persisting lip–tongue dysfunction habit and an unstable cuspal interdigitation after treatment. In general, functional appliances have only a temporary impact on the existing skeletofacial growth pattern. In other words, the inherent morphogenetic pattern dominates over the treatment procedure.

Functional appliances have been shown to be of clinical use in certain cases of hemifacial microsomia. The generation of normal muscle balance in the absence of a condyle results in sufficient bone apposition to restore symmetry. It is speculated that the less severe the deformity, the greater the likelihood of a favorable response. Although it is still controversial, people who have small mandibles may benefit more from functional appliance therapy than patients with normal-sized mandibles.

A functional appliance that is simple and no bulkier than a pair of upper and lower Hawley retainers is the modified Chateau (Great Lakes) appliance. It simply has a wire configuration that comes down from the maxillary Hawley appliance toward the lingual side of the lower incisors and slides down the acrylic of the lower Hawley on the lingual side, thus forcing the mandible into a protruded position. The patient believes that he or she has retainers and does not object to wearing the appliance 24 hours a day. A biteplate could be used as well. The biteplate should not be worn during sleeping hours because the teeth do not contact anyway.

Strong orthopedic forces in the range of 400 to 800 g might be used to reduce a mandibular prognathism with the use of the "chin-cup" appliance. Although a number of significant craniofacial alterations have been noted in patients who underwent orthopedic chin-cup therapy (i.e., retardation of mandibular growth), it seems that a complete inhibition of mandibular growth is difficult to achieve. Growth always continued when a chin cup was worn for 12 to 14 hours per day, which seems to be the greatest practical length of time to expect most patients to wear this appliance. Alteration of the direction was limited to the period that the force was applied. Inherited growth direction seems to be maintained and to recover when the mechanical intervention is removed.

Chin-cup therapy does not necessarily guarantee positive correction of skeletal profile after complete growth, because the skeletal profile is greatly improved during the initial stages of chin-cup therapy but is often not maintained thereafter. To have any permanent results, the patient would have to wear the appliance for many years, well past the completion of growth. Although there have been promising reports in the literature on the combination of chin-cup therapy followed by headgear for vertical control (open-bite cases), the long-term effects of chin-cup therapy for Class-III treatment are still questionable. In addition, although in a recent study it was concluded that chin-cup therapy does not seem to present a functional risk, one cannot ignore the fact that its posteriorly directed force puts a strain on the TMJ (especially if the chin cup is worn for a number of years). The chin-cup appliance needs to be worn well past the cessation of mandibular growth (about 10 years of wear, from 5 to 15 years of age or even more!), something that may not be very practical or easily accepted by the patient. Alternative treatment methods certainly need to be investigated.

Finally, prolonged digit- or pacifier-sucking and tongue-thrusting habits have long been believed to be causative factors in a variety of malocclusions. The most common form of digit sucking is thumb sucking. Graber (1959) points out that three modifying factors—duration, frequency, and intensity—are extremely important and must be recognized and evaluated before the question of damage to the teeth and the tissues is answered. Dental effects include (1) labial inclination or displacement of maxillary incisors with increased overjet, (2) overeruption of posterior teeth, (3) decreased overbite or anterior open bite, (4) linguoversion of mandibular incisors, (5) posterior crossbite, and (6) Class-II molar relation. Skeletal effects include a lowered mandibular posture and autorotation. Spontaneous correction of some components of dental malocclusion is likely if the habit stops by the early mixed dentition.

Tongue thrusting may be defined as an abnormal tongue, perioral, and facial muscle posture and activity during deglutition or at rest. A direct cause-and-effect relation between tongue posture, tongue thrust, swallowing, and malocclusion certainly must be considered. With the increase in overjet that accompanies so many finger-sucking habits, normal swallowing patterns become increasingly difficult. Perioral muscle aberrations, compensatory tongue thrust during swallowing, and abnormal mentalis activity may accelerate the malocclusion.

Treatment for chronic digit sucking and tongue thrusting during the mixed dentition should begin with the simplest form of therapy. For digit-sucking habits, behavior modification may be attempted first, using rewards, encouragement, and reminders. The success of these treatment modalities is judged by both cessation of the habit and significant improvement of the malocclusion. In their article on the effectiveness of various methods of treatment of thumb sucking, Haryett et al. (1967) suggest that palatal crib treatments are more effective than psychological treatment or palatal arch treatment. They also found that most of those treated with the crib stopped the habit in 7 days, and mannerisms did not develop more frequently than in those subjects whose habits had remained active. It should be noted that good rapport with the patient might reduce the incidence of mannerisms and arrest other associated habits. These findings are in accordance with Graber's view that thumb sucking is a simple learned habit (learning theory) without an underlying emotional disturbance.

If the simple attempts fail, then one may try the Thumb Sucking Control Appliance (TCA; GAC International, Central Islip, NY). It can be very easily constructed by bending two to three consecutive loops on a 0.036-inch wire that is designed to fit into the lingual sheaths of the upper first molar bands, just like a regular transpalatal arch. Application minimal chairside time (3–5 minutes), and the appliance can be adjusted to cover the whole span of the patient's open bite, making insertion of the thumb in the mouth very difficult. It is also available in various sizes (preformed).

Bands are fitted on the first maxillary molars and the TCA is inserted late on a Friday afternoon. The child is advised that if he or she quits the habit, the TCA will be removed Monday morning before he or she goes to school, but the bands will be left in place for at least 1 to 2 months. If the habit is initiated again, it is very easy to reinsert the same appliance in the mouth. The child usually complies with this treatment and looks forward to Monday morning. The open bite from the habit should show improvement after cessation of the thumb sucking, within 2 to 4 months. Oral hygiene instructions, along with the recommendation that the parent watch the patient on occasion during sleeping hours to make sure that the patient is not sucking his or her thumb, are part of the therapy plan.

It should be noted that this appliance will work if there is significant overbite and a marked overjet. There must be enough so that it will not interfere with mandibular function. The clinician should be cautioned not to allow the lower incisors to impinge on the wire; otherwise, a functional retrusion would be enhanced.

Often, initiation of fixed appliance therapy (brackets and wires), especially through sutural expansion, results in discontinuation of the habit and in efficient outcomes.

Oral Hygiene

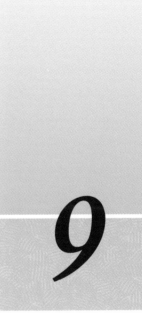

*C*areful inspection at every visit, preventive fluoride programs, and oral hygiene are very important throughout the duration of orthodontic treatment. Proper brushing and flossing three times daily is recommended, followed by fluoride mouth rinses once a day. The combination of daily brushing with a fluoridated dentifrice and daily rinsing with a fluoride wash provides complete protection for the orthodontic patient by inhibiting demineralization or by promoting remineralization of the surfaces at risk. Toothbrushing with a relatively new electric, counterrotational power toothbrush is highly advisable. A rotary electric toothbrush is more effective than conventional toothbrushes for removing plaque and controlling gingivitis in adolescents during orthodontic treatment with fixed appliances. A recent study that compared electric and manual toothbrushing found that the use of the electric system resulted in overall lower plaque scores. Another study of the effectiveness of the new appliance concluded that plaque and gingival scores were significantly lower after brushing for 2 months with the electric counterrotational toothbrush than after brushing with the manual one. Twice-daily use of the Rota-dent electric toothbrush with a standard fluoride toothpaste and once-daily use of a 0.05% NaF rinse is more effective for preventing decalcification in adolescents during orthodontic treatment with fixed appliances than either conventional toothbrushing with a fluoride toothpaste, or toothbrushing and toothpaste with a once-daily NaF rinse. Electric toothbrushes of the new generation are a real alternative to the often laborious manual tooth cleaning procedure used during active appliance therapy. Patients with poor oral hygiene may benefit from their use especially because plaque removal can be achieved easier and faster. The orthodontic treatment itself has an impact on oral hygiene in the long term as well; a study showed that children who received orthodontic treatment had a greater reduction of plaque and gingivitis than children who did not. This was related more to behavior factors than to improved tooth alignment.

Orthodontic treatment during adolescence has no discernible effect on late periodontal health. In the absence of compromising conditions, adult patients are not inherently more likely than adolescents to lose dental support during treatment. The adult patient should visit the periodontist every 3 to 4 months for check-ups. The use of motivational techniques and a specific mission and philosophy within a private orthodontic practice can help reduce total treatment time.

Good oral hygiene by the patient may also contribute to reduced treatment time.

Oral rinses, such as Listerine, can be effective adjuncts if compliance is good. Cases with unmanageable gingival inflammation can be put on a 6-week regimen of rinsing with Peridex twice daily. Ibuprofen is a preferred analgesic in the treatment of discomfort because of postorthodontic adjustments. Patients are advised to brush, floss (with Superfloss), and rinse with Listerine, and then with fluoride.

Treatment

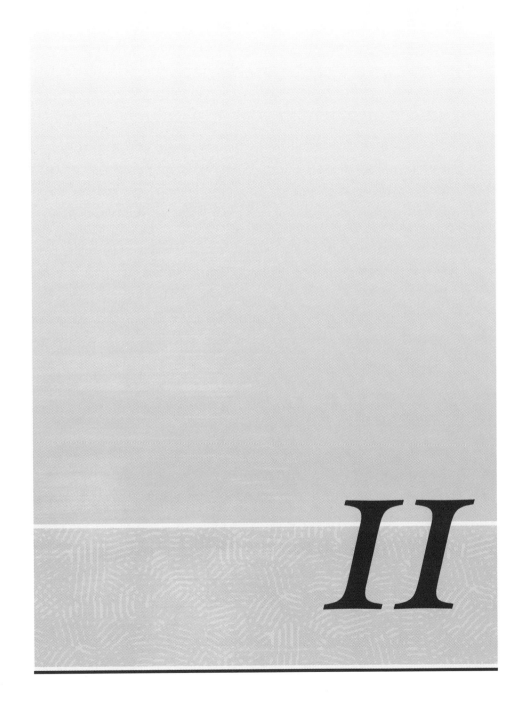

II

Tooth Movement Simplified

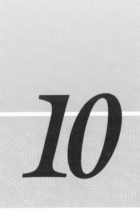

According to Creekmore (1982), in orthodontics, we need less force with greater tooth movements. The first place to start this quest is in the selection of the bracket that is attached to the teeth. If this is overlooked or underestimated, then the greatest mistake has already been made (Figures 44–46).

The new superelastic wires provide less force and greater tooth movements. The stainless steel wires, no matter what their size, could not do this. The superelastic nickel-titanium alloy archwire (NiTi) was found to give improved alignment compared with the more traditional, multiple-stranded steel archwire. This difference was found to be statistically significant only in the region of the lower labial segment.

The superelastic wires allow us to use even square or rectangular wires as initial archwires for total tooth movement (crown and root). Thus, the bracket design should be such that it maximizes the potential of the multifunctional superelastic wires from the onset of therapy (Figures 47–50).

The maximum potential of any archwire is achieved when we use the largest-size wire possible (Figures 51–57). Therefore, we would need maximum interslot distance for maximum archwire flexibility to be able to engage a large archwire in the bracket slot (Figure 58).

If x is the length of the wire between the slots of two adjacent twin (square) brackets, then the distance between the slots of a triangular bracket (Bioefficient; OrthoSystems Inc., Plano, TX) with a single-slot (narrow) bracket would be $1.5x$ (Figures 59, 60). Because stiffness is inversely proportional to the cube of the length of the wire $(\frac{1}{x})^3$ and the amount of deflection or range is proportional to the square of the length of the wire (x^2), then an archwire between narrow-slot brackets would have 3.37 times less stiffness and 2.25 times greater activation, and thus overall much greater flexibility. It is obvious, then, that single-slot brackets (narrow) would be more efficient. Then why have they not been as popular as the twin systems available? The answer to this is because the narrow-width (single-type) brackets have virtually no rotational capability or tipping control (Figures 61–64).

Based on the writings of Schwartz at the beginning of this century, the "father" of fixed and edgewise orthodontics, Dr. Edward Angle, used a rigid archwire termed the "E" arch. The "E" stood for "expansion." Teeth were pulled out to the "E" archwire with ligature wires. The archwire was not meant originally to be deflected to the teeth. In the early 1900s Dr. Angle and his disciples could use any material for archwires, provided it was a gold alloy. Stainless steel was not used in orthodontics until the 1930s. The gold archwire size selected by Dr. Angle measured 0.022 by 0.036 inches. Initially, the 0.036-inch dimension was occlusogingival or placed as a ribbon arch.

In 1925, Dr. Angle proposed the "Edgewise" appliance. By placing the 0.022 by 0.036-inch ribbon arch on edge, rather than "flatwise" to the teeth, and with the use of a bracket with an edgewise rectangular slot, Dr. Angle could apply the moments of force in all three planes. Further refinements followed, and the gold alloy edgewise archwire was reduced in size to 0.022 by 0.025 inches.

In the 1940s, stainless steel replaced gold alloys for orthodontic appliances. Up until then, all fixed appliances (edgewise) used a 0.022-inch bracket slot. With the use of stainless steel, which is about 20% stiffer than gold alloy, orthodontists could afford to use a smaller-diameter wire and still deliver the same force as the less stiff, larger gold alloy. Hence, the 0.018-inch slot could be used, which is 20% smaller than the 0.022-inch slot. Thus, we now have two sizes of edgewise bracket slots and a wide variety of wires to match. The 0.022-inch size was arrived at empirically in the early 1900s, and the 0.018-inch size was the result of a materials change based on the same original empiricism, not on any new insights in biomechanics.

In the 1990s, full-size, rectangular archwires are available that deliver less force than small-diameter, round stainless steel. Are these newer titanium alloys as effective and efficient at tooth movement? This question raises a great many issues. A fundamental issue is that of optimum force levels for efficient and biologically acceptable tooth movement. A general trend toward lower force levels seems to be taking place. Forces delivered to individual teeth in the 1920s were likely in the range of hundreds of grams. A titanium alloy archwire, deflected to the most severely malapposed tooth in an arch, is measured in tens of grams. Yet, teeth seem to be moving just as rapidly, if not more so. Most believe, at least intuitively, that light, continuous forces are physiologically more acceptable than heavier, intermittent forces. If this premise has some truth to it, then why not use the lightest force that will get the job done within a reasonable treatment time?

The introduction of the superelastic wires has led to clinical applications hitherto unfeasible in patient care. These wires are very different from the first-generation work-hardened NiTi wires (M-NiTi) and, of course, the stainless steel wires, in that they possess shape memory and superelastic properties. The release rates of nickel or chromium from stainless steel and nickel-titanium arch wires are not significantly different. Orthodontic treatment does not seem to increase the risk for nickel hypersensitivity. There may be a risk of sensitizing patients to nickel with long-term exposure to nickel-containing appliances, as occurs in routine orthodontic therapy. The biodegradation of orthodontic appliances during the initial 5 months of treatment did not result in significant or consistent increases in the blood level of nickel. The superelastic properties of NiTi alloy wires and their use in osteoclast recruitment represent a significant scientific breakthrough for orthodontics. Their use should establish a new standard of biologic treatment in orthodontics. Regardless of the extent of activation, these wires provide a light, constant force at oral temperatures (superelasticity). Before wire insertion in the brackets, the clinician may use local ice application or preserve them in the refrigerator. This decreased temperature allows them to be in their "plastic phase" (martensinic), where they can be easily placed into the bracket slots. At oral temperatures (austensinic), they resume their original arch-form shape (shape memory) (Figures 65–68).

The combination of shape memory and superelasticity makes these wires very comfortable for the patient, even in a rectangular form when used as initial archwires (Figures 69, 70). The nonlinear unloading of these wires has an initial rapid drop in the force level applied to the teeth, which implies that less force is applied on larger activation. The wire stiffness increases and the wire becomes more effective toward the end of movement, and thus the clinician should not be too hasty in changing the wire or seeing the patient too often. A 2-month appointment interval is well justified for such wire activation (Figures 71–77). One must be very careful not to apply excess finger pressure for wire engagement because exceeding the deformation limit of the superelastic wire would cause very high forces that may lead to unwanted side effects (Figures 78–85).

Because these wires are temperature sensitive (heat-activated wires), the clinician may choose to advise his or her patients to alternate a hot meal with a cold drink on a daily basis. Theoretically, the cold drink will return wires to their "plastic," martensinic phase, and thus perhaps allow them momentarily to self-adjust in the bracket slots as the teeth move between appointments. The hot meal will quickly bring the mouth temperature to the activation temperature for these wires. If nothing else, these wires involve patients in their treatment because they feel they activate or "energize" their own appliances and thus actively participate in the final outcome.

The low moduli of elasticity of the newer orthodontic alloys permit the use of light, rectangular or square wires even during the early stages of treatment. Rectangular or square wires are preferable over round wires because they can be oriented in the bracket in such a way that forces work out in the proper directions. They maintain better control over root position by delivering both movements and forces. The use of stainless steel wires only to treat an entire case from start to finish may be indicated only in relatively few patients. It may be beneficial instead to exploit the desirable qualities of a particular wire type that is specifically selected to satisfy the demands of the presenting clinical situation. This would provide the most optimal and efficient treatment results.

The superelastic rectangular or square wires allow for initial full bracket engagement for correction of rotations, alignment, initial leveling, and space closure. Thus, in contemporary orthodontics, the clinician may approach the first three stages of orthodontic therapy (alignment, leveling, space closure) as part I of treatment, and finishing as part II. This immediately preconditions the clinician to spend an equal amount of time finishing a case (one half the total treatment time vs. one fourth, as was thought previously). In most cases, a two-wire system is used: the initial archwire is a superelastic wire (round or rectangular) and the finishing wire is stainless steel (round or rectangular). The objective is to start alignment, leveling, and space closure with the superelastic wires and finish with the stainless steel wires. Every attempt should be made to place the stainless steel wires as soon as possible if leveling is to be enhanced.

It should be emphasized that the objective of the mechanotherapy is to make the transition toward the finishing stainless steel wire as soon as possible (within 4 to 6 months). Although any space closure may have started on the superelastic wire, it is frequently finished with the stainless steel one. A 10° toe-in may be added in the wire distal to the second premolars to prevent mesial molar rotation. Although the lower incisor brackets have a −5° torque that positions the lower incisor roots forward to increase anterior anchorage, it may become necessary to add a 10° anterior lingual crown torque to the stainless steel wire to increase the anchorage, especially if Class-II elastics are used over an extended period of time (> 4 months). A slight reverse curve of Spee may also be necessary in the mandibular arch to counteract the extrusive effect on the molar from the elastics. When the posterior segment needs to be protracted, this should be done sequentially (one tooth at a time) with a 10° to 20° anterior labial crown torque added to the wire. In addition, a NiTi uprighting spring may be added through the vertical slot of the cuspid brackets to move the crown anteriorly to increase the anterior anchorage and minimize its tendency toward posterior tooth protraction.

Because of the wide range of activation of superelastic wires, the clinician may see some patients for adjustments every 8 to 12 weeks—in other words, every 2 to 3 months! Of course, the superelastic wire can be reactivated on a monthly basis by simply untying it from the bracket slot and retying it back in. This returns the force level to the original activated state, which may expedite tooth movement at still lower levels of force. The patient and parent need to be educated on the advances in material technology and thus appreciate the service they are receiving. Doctor's time is greatly reduced, and the number of patients that can be seen is greater than in years past.

It should be pointed out that there is a significant difference in the flexibility of the rectangular wires, for example, a 0.018 by 0.025-inch difference between activation in the vertical versus the horizontal plane. This means that it is much easier to engage a high cuspid in a wire on its vertical activation of 5 to 7 mm than to engage the wire fully into the bracket slot of a tooth that needs to be rotated 2 to 3 mm. This is because the dimension of the wire in the vertical plane (0.018 inch) is less than that in the horizontal plane (0.025 inch). This is why, when severe rotations are present, it may be preferable to use a round or square superelastic wire instead of a rectangular one, because the dimensions of such wires are the same in both the vertical and horizontal planes. Rectangular or square wires are used from the start of therapy as initial wires in cases where simultaneous alignment of the crown and roots is desired (extensive root movement). Round wires are used in cases where dental compensations need be maintained.

The evolution of the superelastic wires began with the introduction of the round Sentalloy (GAC) wires. These are available in light, medium, and heavy forces. The rectangular series, under the name Neo Sentalloy, followed at 100, 200, and 300 g. Later, the rectangular and square Bioforce wires were introduced that demonstrated 80 g of force in the central incisor region for tooth alignment and up to 320 g in the molar region for efficient posterior leveling. Recently, the new Bioforce Ionguard wire was introduced. Ionguard is a nitrogen layer that covers the top 3 μm of the superelastic nickel-titanium wires after ion bombardment of the wire surface. This wire seems to demonstrate less friction, breakage, and nickel release because of the manufacturing process. It is the author's choice for an initial archwire because it is the most versatile wire for initiation of simultaneous alignment, leveling, and space closure. Other wires have recently been introduced that are more or less similar to the original superelastics. None of them demonstrate the progressive increase in force delivery levels within the same wire (from anterior 80 g to posterior 320 g) as the Bioforce wire. The impact of differential force delivery within the same wire for anterior alignment and posterior leveling is obvious.

Tie-back with superelastic materials can be accomplished through a crimpable hook placed directly on the archwire in front of the molar tooth. The hooks may slide on to the archwire and can be secured into position with crimping pliers. Even if the second molar is not included in the main archwire (although this is highly recommended), a wire-tie should connect a bonded attachment on this tooth to the first molar for additional anchorage. The superelastic wire may also be heated posteriorly and bent behind the molar tube. A step may also be placed with step-pliers to avoid sliding of the wire on one side owing to less friction in the triangular brackets (Bioefficient).

The superelastic wires cannot be conformed in the transverse dimension. At present, they are available only in two or three archforms. No single archform is ideal for every patient, and each archwire requires individualization to produce the best overall result. This is why the finishing stainless steel wires should be placed as soon as possible and conformed to the patient's original mandibular arch. Individualization of the orthodontic archform for each patient is highly recommended.

Figures 44–46

In the past, multilooped wires, big, bulky brackets, and uncomfortable bands would result in tissue irritation, pain on activation, and a very displeasing appearance.

Figure 44

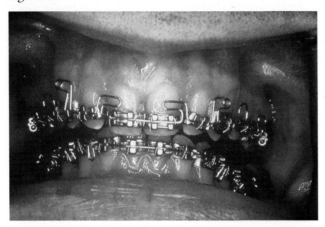

Figure 45

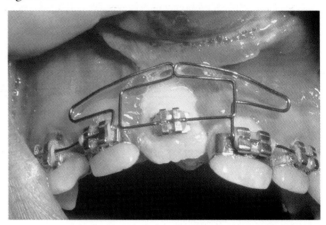

Figure 46

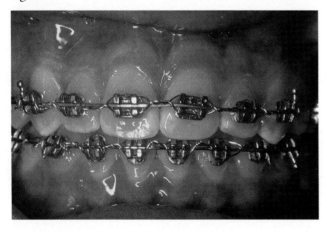

Figures 47–50

Today's triangular (Bioefficient) brackets (OrthoSystem Inc., Plano, TX) not only provide more room for activation of the new, flexible, heat-activated nickel-titanium (NiTi) wires compared with the twin (square) brackets (compare the left side of Figure 48 with the right), but result in faster tooth movement because of less friction in the bracket. These canines were brought into alignment in just 6 months of treatment with just one square flexible wire (20 × 20 Bioforce Ionguard [GAC International] in a 0.022-inch slot). The amount of force needed to move teeth is very low, approximately 0.025 g/cm^2, the same as the blood pressure in the capillaries. Higher force levels will cause "hyalinization" or "temporary necrosis" of the surrounding tissues, which takes about 7 to 14 days to reorganize. Pain occurs as well. The forces applied with the stainless steel wires are always heavier than needed, thus causing a delay period of 7 to 14 days with no tooth movement. During this time, undermining resorption occurs (from within the bone) until it reaches the bone surface after 7 to 14 days, at which point the bone is reabsorbed and the tooth is moved abruptly. Hyalinization occurs again, and so on. This happens even with the lightest stainless steel wires (i.e., 0.012 inch). The superelastic NiTi wires can be displaced a considerable distance without developing excessive force, and they return to their original position because of shape memory. The Bioforce wire also delivers lighter forces in the front and heavier in the back (for the bigger teeth). Shape memory refers to the phenomenon in which the alloy is soft and readily amenable to change in shape at a low temperature, but can easily be reformed to its original configuration when it is heated to a suitable transition temperature. The superelastic property is demonstrated when the stress value remains fairly constant up to a certain point of wire deformation and, as the wire deformation rebounds, the stress value again remains fairly constant. This NiTi wire possesses all of the aforementioned properties and can therefore deliver a relatively constant force for a long period of time, which is considered a physiologically desirable force for tooth movement. This new NiTi alloy exerts an extremely light, continuous force, regardless of deflection, and this superelastic force can be applied at low levels, regardless of wire size. The rectangular or square NiTi wires have excellent clinical application, especially in the early phases of orthodontic treatment (i.e., alignment and leveling). The rectangular or square NiTi wires can replace all stainless steel round wires, as well as some of the rectangular ones, but not the finishing stainless steel wires that are necessary for fine detailing, arch coordination, and finishing bends. By using rectangular archwires from the onset of treatment, torque control is immediately obtained. This may be important in posttreatment stability. In addition, canine retraction can be initiated from the onset of treatment. By the time the canine teeth are in a solid Class-I relationship (about 5 months into treatment, figures 49, 50), alignment and leveling have been completed and the patient is ready to receive the stainless steel finishing coordinated archwires, which will be the final archwires of therapy.

Figure 47

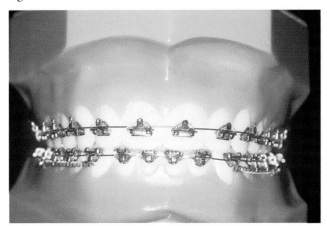

Figure 48

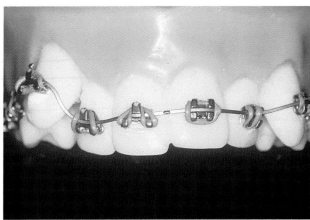

Figure 49

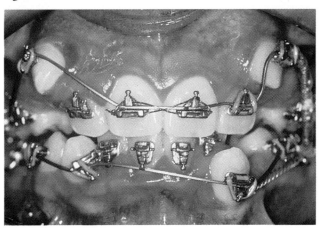

Figure 50

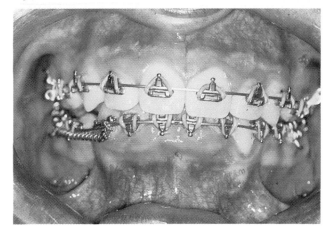

Figure 51

There are three general shapes of orthodontic wires: round, square, and rectangular. Even though in the past most of these wires were made of stainless steel, the development of NiTi wires has led to the wide range of "elastic" wires that are available today.

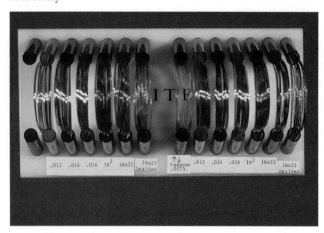

Figure 52

Conventional orthodontic mechanotherapy has four steps of treatment: alignment, leveling, space closure, and finishing. Each phase of treatment would last about 6 months to a year, for a total treatment time of 2 to 3 years for most cases.

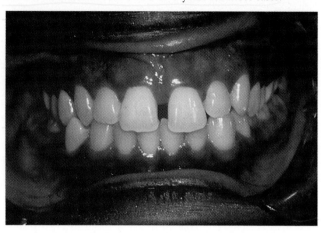

Figures 53–55

In the past, both alignment and leveling were done simultaneously with light, round, stainless steel wires with monthly progression to a larger-diameter wire. This sequence in the 0.018-inch slot system is 0.012-inch, followed by 0.014-inch, and then 0.016-inch diameter round wires. The objective was to start with a very fine wire, such as 0.012-inch wire, that would have the least stiffness (stiffness is a measure of the amount of force required to bend a wire a certain distance), so that it may be fully engaged in the bracket slot without deformation and thus start tooth movement with the least discomfort to the patient. If even lighter force levels were needed, braided stainless steel archwires could also be used. Usually, as the teeth would have moved toward the correct archform, the next size wire would be inserted in the brackets. One must remember that the stiffer the wire, the more force it takes to place it in the bracket, and thus, the more force it will deliver and the more pain it will elicit. This is a time-consuming and sometimes painful process.

Figure 53

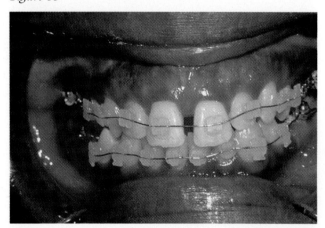

Figure 54

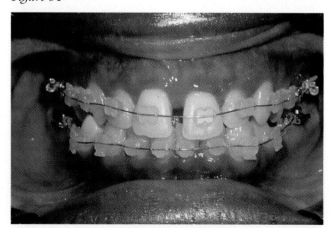

Figures 53–55 (continued)

Figure 55

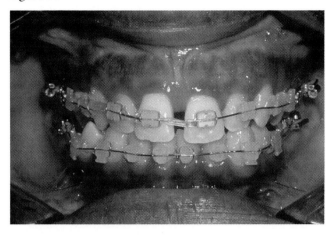

Figures 56, 57

Space closure in the 0.018-inch slot system would begin with a 0.016 × 0.016-inch rectangular stainless steel wire, followed by a 0.016 × 0.022-inch wire. The finishing archwire would be a 0.016 × 0.022-inch wire or a 0.017 × 0.025-inch wire. In the 0.022-inch slot, the finishing archwire is usually a 0.019 × 0.025-inch wire.

Figure 56

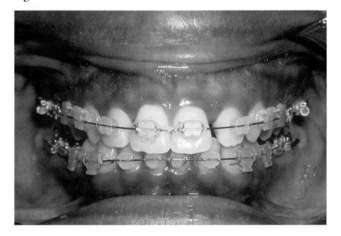

Figure 57

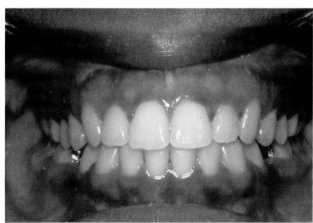

Figure 58

The triangular brackets provide a lot of room for initial arch-wire engagement regardless of tooth position. Mouth temperature straightens out the wire, ultimately bringing the teeth into their proper position in the arch. The clinician needs to see the patient only every 2 to 3 months because the movement is no longer mechanically induced with stainless steel wires, as in years past. Instead, movement is biologically induced, because the wire is manufactured to straighten out when warmed to mouth temperature.

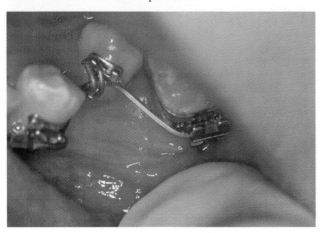

Figure 59

The new triangular brackets are twin brackets (bottom half) with a single-slot type (upper half). The slot is elevated so that the wire may come in contact with the side elbow extensions during movement (similar to a "see-saw") and thus provide for differential levels of wire stiffness during movement. The vertical slot is used primarily to tie the wire onto the flexed main archwire if insertion in the actual slot is, for whatever reason, not possible.

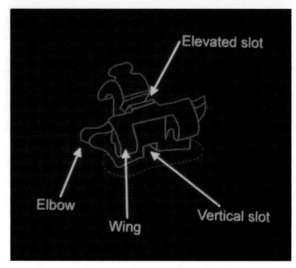

Figure 60

The triangular bracket (Bioefficient) was designed to provide the first differential stiffness bracket to accommodate the new, differential-force superelastic wire (Bioforce). On insertion of the wire in the brackets, the large interslot distance allows for maximum wire flexibility (low stiffness). On maximum movement, especially in the direction opposite to adjacent teeth, the interelbow distance ensures minimum flexibility of the same initial wire (high stiffness) for immediate control. Most of the movements are accomplished on the elbow–slot distance, which is still smaller than the interbracket of a conventional twin bracket. Thus, the triangular bracket allows for easier wire insertion than a twin (square) bracket and even better control during movement.

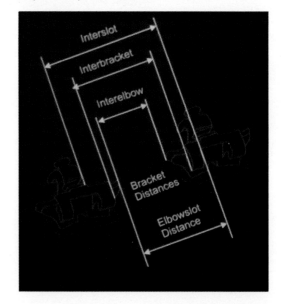

Figures 61, 62

Most conventional single-slot brackets provide inadequate tip control during movement, resulting in unnecessary round-tipping of teeth and waste of treatment time.

Figure 61

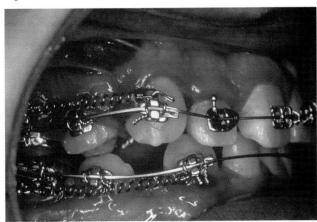

Figure 62

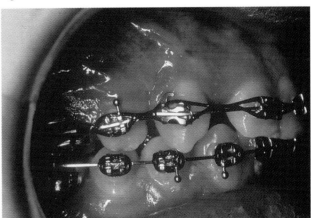

Figures 63, 64

Even small twin (square) brackets do not control tip very well because the interslot distance is too great. In this case, it took an additional treatment time of 3 months to upright these teeth.

Figure 63

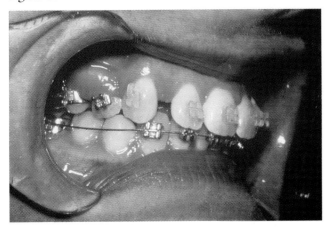

Figure 64

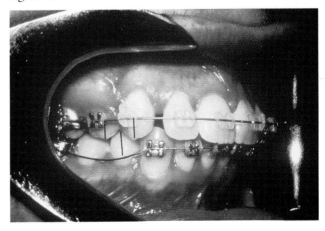

Figure 65

Insertion of the new superelastic wire in the triangular brackets. Note the distance between the slots versus the wings of these brackets. There is much more room between these brackets for wire insertion compared with conventional twin brackets.

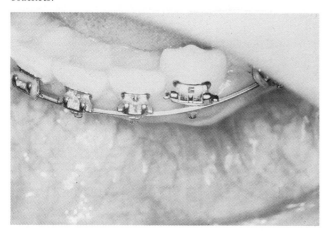

Figure 66

The wire is cooled with a frozen cotton roll for 10 seconds.

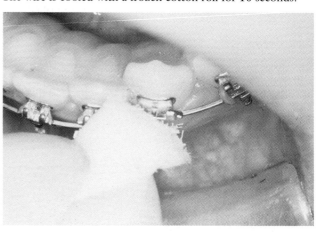

Figure 67

The wire becomes soft under cold temperatures and enters the interslot distance with gentle finger pressure. Note the gentle flow of the wire from the lateral incisor bracket to the canine.

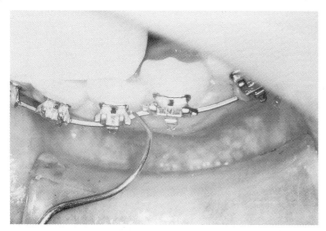

Figure 68

The elastomeric module simply holds the wire in place. As the wire warms up with mouth temperature, it will straighten the canine.

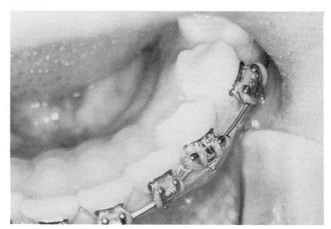

Figure 69

Activation of the wire in another patient. Note the gentle flow of the wire from bracket to bracket. The wire does not have to be fully in the slot; it simply must "flow." The elastomeric module holds it. As the wire warms up to mouth temperature, it will move the tooth.

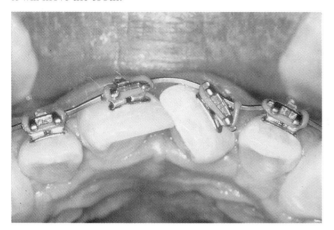

Figure 70

The same patient just 2 months later. Note the significant correction that has already taken place. The whole system works like windsurfing: the module just holds on to the wire as the "sail" turns and moves.

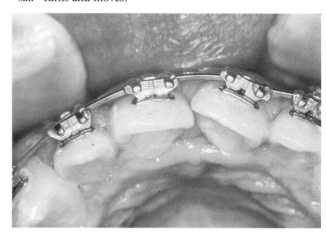

Figure 71

Same patient as in Figures 69 and 70 with severe rotation of the upper incisor.

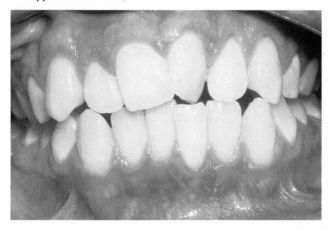

Figure 72

After maxillary sutural expansion for 1 month, the 20 × 20 Bioforce Ionguard wire is placed in the 0.022-inch slot triangular brackets (compare this picture to Figure 69).

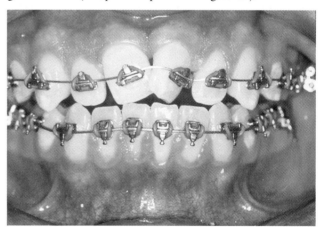

Figure 73

Two months later, note the significant rotation and root up-righting of the central incisor (compare with Figure 70).

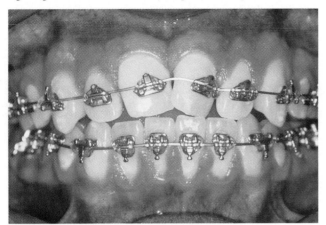

Figure 74

Four months into treatment, the incisors are almost upright.

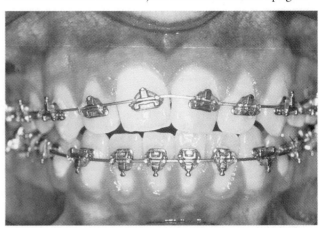

Figure 75

Six months into treatment, the teeth are well aligned in the arch.

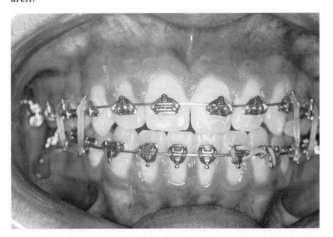

Figure 76

Eight months into treatment, elastics are used to obtain inter-cuspation. The same initial wires are still in place.

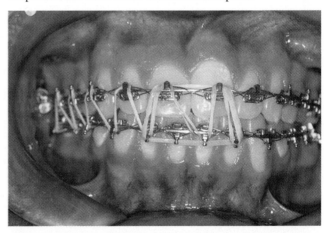

Section II: *Treatment*

Figure 77

Ten months into treatment, the case is almost completed. Note the beautiful intercuspation, canine position, and midline correction. This case would have taken much longer with stainless steel mechanics.

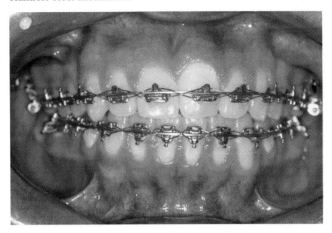

Figure 78

Patient with conventional twin (square) brackets on the upper incisors. Note that the upper left lateral incisors cannot be fully engaged using a superelastic rectangular wire.

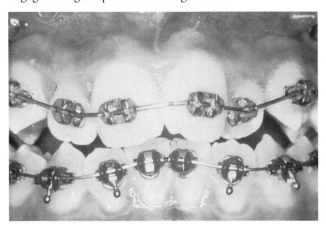

Figure 79

Two months later, gentle finger pressure still cannot engage the wire in the mesial wing of the bracket after the wire has been cooled. At this point, significant finger pressure was applied to the wire for full engagement.

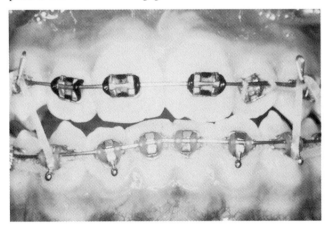

Figures 80, 81

Radiographs before and after treatment of the patient in Figures 78 and 79. Note the iatrogenic root resorption that was induced from the finger pressure referred to in Figure 79. At the time, the clinician was unaware of it. Too much finger pressure, customary with stainless steel mechanics, is unacceptable with the new wire technology because it dramatically increases the level of forces the moment the deformation of the wire is more than 8%. Therefore, only temperature change should be allowed to deform the wire, with gentle finger pressure. This is why the triangular brackets are more appropriate for the new wire technology, because they allow for maximum interslot distance and a gentle "flow" of the wire from bracket to bracket.

Figure 80

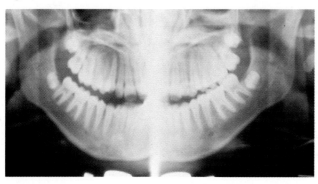

Figure 81

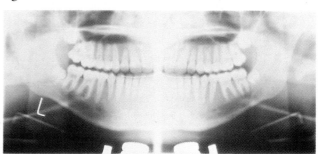

Figure 82

This patient has triangular brackets. The upper first premolars were extracted because of the crowding and maxillary procumbency. The wire was inserted at this first appointment after the brackets were attached on to the teeth. (Courtesy of Drs. Janson, Martins, Henriques, de Freitas, Pinzan, and de Almeida of the University of São Paulo, Bauru Dental School, Brazil.)

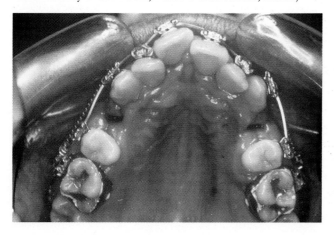

Figure 83

Two months later! The spaces are almost completely closed and the teeth already well aligned. The patient was comfortable. (Courtesy of Drs. Janson, Martins, Henriques, de Freitas, Pinzan, and de Almeida of the University of São Paulo, Bauru Dental School, Brazil.)

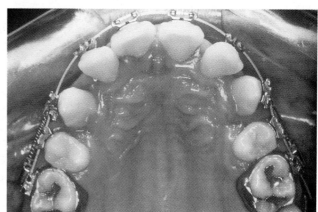

The roots of the teeth that moved are beautifully aligned. Fast movement with light forces induced biologically from mouth temperature, with almost no friction from the triangular brackets (see Section II, Chapter 14), allow for fast and easy tooth movement. (Courtesy of Drs. Janson, Martins, Henriques, de Freitas, Pinzan, and de Almeida of the University of São Paulo, Bauru Dental School, Brazil.)

Figure 84

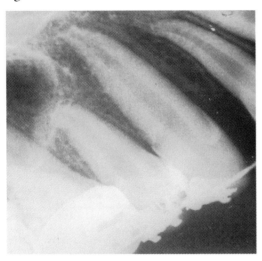

Figure 85

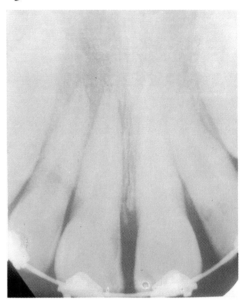

Archwire Sequence

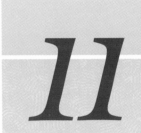

The introduction of superelastic wires in orthodontics has brought about the clinical realization that it is not archwire size that determines the incorporation of wires in the bracket slots, but the actual interslot distance. As the large interslot distance of the new orthodontic brackets increases, the flexibility of the superelastic orthodontic wires allows the clinician to start with large, round, square, or even rectangular archwires as initial ones from the beginning of treatment (see Figures 65–70). The objective of the wire sequence would be to maximize the effectiveness and use the versatility of these wires for initial simultaneous alignment, leveling, and space closure (see Figures 71–77). The following is a recommended archwire sequence that is based on superelastic and stainless steel wires.

0.022-inch Slot

Most clinicians in the 0.022-inch system finish with a 0.019×0.025-inch stainless steel wire. This wire should be engaged as soon as possible in the bracket slots to expeditiously finish the leveling and space closure processes and detail the occlusion.

Thus, the focus of initial mechanotherapy should be the efficient transition to finishing 0.019×0.025-inch stainless steel archwire. In other words, the initial wire of choice should be versatile enough to allow the incorporation of the finishing wire as soon as possible as the second and final wire of treatment. This is accomplished nicely if we use a starting archwire that is larger than the final one.

The archwire that is larger than the 0.019×0.025-inch size is the 0.020×0.020-inch square one. The square shape of the wire allows for adequate control of torque and tip and the incorporation of most malaligned teeth in both the vertical and horizontal dimensions.

Surprisingly enough, the 0.020×0.020-inch superelastic square wire may be incorporated as the initial archwire in most cases with great ease in brackets with a large interslot distance, especially with local ice treatment to cool the wire down to its plastic phase. Its large, square shape gives the clinician the necessary control to initiate leveling and space closure at the same time that alignment is taking place. It does not fill the slot completely, and thus friction between the bracket slot and the wire is minimized. At the same time, it brings the bracket slots in such a relation that the 0.019 × 0.025-inch finishing stainless steel wire may be engaged much earlier in treatment than a smaller wire in one dimension (the 0.022 inch).

Thus, it is the opinion of this author that the most efficient archwire sequence for most cases in the 0.022 bracket slot system is the following two-wire sequence:

Initial wire: 0.020 × 0.020-inch superelastic wire

Finishing wire: 0.019 × 0.025-inch stainless wire

On a similar note, the clinician may start with an 0.018 × 0.025-inch superelastic rectangular Bioforce Ionguard wire and finish with the 0.019 × 0.025-inch stainless steel wire. In this case, although the initial wire is not larger in either dimension, it is of equal size in one (the 0.025 inch) and only slightly smaller in the other (0.018 vs. 0.019 inch). This is also another efficient archwire sequence that clinicians may use with the 0.022-inch slot system.

0.018-inch Slot

In the 0.018-inch bracket slot system, the finishing archwires of choice for most clinicians seem to be the 0.016 × 0.022-inch or the 0.017 × 0.025-inch stainless steel rectangular or square wires. Thus, if we were to follow the aforementioned thoughts, the initial archwire of choice with superelastic properties would be the 0.018 × 0.018-inch square or 0.018 × 0.025-inch rectangular wires. Notice that the size of both of these wires brings at least one side of the wire (the 0.018-inch side) in full contact with the bracket slot, and thus friction is enhanced. As a result, some of the earlier work on patients in the 0.018 slot system used the 0.016 × 0.022-inch superelastic wire as the initial wire. In other words, even though the 0.018 × 0.025-inch superelastic wire can be readily engaged in brackets of a large interslot distance, the limited freedom of movement (because of friction in both dimensions) along the archwire may not make it the most efficient wire in cases requiring extensive tooth movement (as compared with the 0.018 × 0.018-inch square wire).

On the other hand, if wires made with the Ionguard process (nitrogen substitution of top 3 μm of nickel of wire surface) are used, such friction is greatly reduced. Thus, one may use the 0.018 × 0.025-inch rectangular superelastic wires as initial archwires without too much friction and with excellent tip and torque control.

Therefore, it is this author's opinion that the most efficient archwire sequence in the 0.018-inch slot system is:

Initial archwire: 0.018 × 0.018 or 0.016 × 0.022 or 0.018 × 0.025-inch superelastic wire

Finishing archwire: 0.017 × 0.025-inch or 0.016 × 0.022-inch stainless wire

Bracket Prescription

12

*I*f one were to observe closely an ideal dental arch, it would immediately become apparent that the position of each tooth in the alveolus is defined by three parameters: (1) the "in-out" position, (2) the crown angulation or "tip," and (3) the crown inclination, or "torque." These three parameters define the three-dimensional position of each tooth in its space. In the past, all orthodontic brackets were the same for all teeth, with the same slot. The clinician had to incorporate into the main archwire three bends for each tooth to maneuver each tooth in its ideal position: (1) the "in-out" or first-order bend, (2) the "tip" or second-order bend, and (3) the "torque" or third-order bend. Modern fixed appliances have all these bends built into their slots, making each bracket specific for each tooth. Providing that the bracket is positioned ideally on the tooth surface (in the middle of the crown, along the long axis, and parallel to the incisal edge), these preadjusted prescription appliances theoretically have the capability to finish the treatment with no bends in the archwires whatsoever! Obviously, this is like saying that everyone's feet should fit in the same size shoe. No matter how perfect bracket placement is with preadjusted appliances, compensating bends or bracket repositioning are always needed at the end of treatment for final detailing and finishing of the occlusion.

All suggested numbers in the following recommended prescription are aimed at overcorrecting the malocclusion and working with large-size archwires from the onset of treatment. It should be emphasized that it is impossible to "fit everybody into the same size shoe." Full-size or undersized wires should be used accordingly, and individual finishing is almost always required.

Bracket Prescription

Upper Central Incisor

First-order bend (in-out): **Standard**
Second-order bend (tip): **5°**
Third-order bend (torque): **20°**

A specific thickness is given to the upper incisor bracket of a regular size. A 5° angulation is similar to the one proposed by Andrews (1972) in his classic work. It is also widely used in other prescriptions. The 20° torque is definitely greater than the torque proposed by Andrews (1972), Roth (1985), and Alexander (1986), and close to the 22° suggested by Hilgers (1987). Because sliding mechanics are used, it would be quite easy to "dump" the anterior teeth lingually during retraction and space closure. Accentuated torque would reduce this, and by the end of treatment the teeth would be positioned similarly to what Andrews proposed for the ideal occlusion (7°). In addition, it is easier to alleviate the torque effect by using undersized rectangular or square wires than by adding torque in the wire. Because 0.001 inch of play (tolerance) relates to approximately 4° of torque lost, a finishing 0.019×0.025-inch stainless steel wire would allow 12° of torque effect lost, if desired in the 0.022 slot. In the 0.018 slot, the finishing archwire of 0.016×0.022 inch is also undersized. If no expression of the prescription is desired, then a large round wire may be used, maintaining the dental compensations.

Upper Lateral Incisor

First-order bend (in-out): **Greater thickness**

Second-order bend (tip): **10°**

Third-order bend (torque): **10°**

Greater bracket thickness is needed to compensate for the buccal–lingual relation of the lateral incisor compared with the central incisor. The 10° angulation is slightly greater than that suggested by Andrews (1972) and Roth (1985) (9°) or Alexander (1986) and Hilgers (1987) (8°), but similar to that recommended by Ricketts (1981) (10°). This additional angulation is needed to prevent close proximity of the central and lateral incisor roots, especially during space closure. The 10° torque is again greater than that in other prescriptions for the same reasons addressed for the central incisor bracket.

Upper Cuspid

First-order bend (in-out): **Thinner than central incisor**

Second-order bend (tip): **10°**

Third-order bend (torque): **5°**

The bracket thickness on the cuspid has to be thinner than the regular size of the upper central incisor because of the bulkiness of the cuspid. The 10° of tip are similar to that proposed by Roth (1985) (13°) without positioning the root of the tooth too distally and still enhancing bodily movement and reducing the tipping effect of sliding mechanics with anchorage loss. A 5° torque is necessary because, as supported by Hilgers (1987), there is a mechanical tendency to detorque the upper canines as they are retracted in extraction cases, and there is always the possibility of impacting the root on the dense cortical labial plate on space closure. In nonextraction cases, where a slight expansion occurs in all cases and the tooth is tipped outward, the effect of the torque can be minimized by placing an undersized finishing wire (i.e., a 0.016×0.022-inch wire in the 0.018 slot system or 0.019×0.025-inch in the 0.022 slot system).

High lingual torque on the upper cuspid is also advocated in the prescriptions of Hilgers and Ricketts to maintain the integrity of the labial surface contours between the cuspid and the lateral by keeping their torque differential to a minimum. In addition, a more vertical inclination of the upper canines alleviates the detrimental effects of the "narrow cuspid" look, which is also detrimental to functional jaw movements and the periodontal health of the tissues overlying prominent roots. Thus, a nice, broad "Hollywood"-type smile is created with a gentle rise in excursions and stability through reduction of excessive lateral forces.

Upper Premolars

First-order bend (in-out): **Similar to the cuspid**

Second-order bend (tip): **0°**

Third-order bend (torque): **5°**

The first-order compensation is the same as that for the cuspid because of their similar prominence. The 0° tip agrees with the overcorrected position suggested in most prescriptions. The −5° torque placed on the premolars, although it encourages "dropping down" of the lingual cusps, does so just enough to ensure good intercuspation of the bicuspid teeth with their counterparts of the opposing arch. This comes as the result of numerous observations of finished cases that appeared fine from the buccal side but from the lingual side lacked the nice, solid occlusion of an ideally finished case. Undersized wires can be used in openbite tendency cases.

Upper Molars

First-order bend (in-out): **Very thin mesially/thick distally (20°)**

Second-order bend (tip): **0°**

Third-order bend (torque): **−10°**

As suggested by Hilgers (1987), a 20° distal rotation of this tooth ensures the shortest arch length occupied by the first molar tooth, which is 5° more than Andrews' recommendation. Thus, the bracket should be very thin around the mesiobuccal cusp and very thick on the distobuccal cusp. A 20° distal overrotation is especially helpful in the overcorrection of Class-II, division 1 cases, and it counteracts the movements placed on the molar teeth from the side effects of sliding mechanotherapy. The 0° angulation is similar to other prescriptions. The −10° torque allows for a good intercuspal occlusion, especially of the lingual cusps.

Lower Incisors

First-order bend (in-out): **Thick**

Second-order bend (tip): **0°**

Third-order bend (torque): **−5°**

Thick brackets on the lower incisors compensate for their lingual relation relative to the upper anteriors. The 0° tip positions these teeth in an upright position, whereas the −5° torque, similar to that suggested by Alexander (1986), has been shown to hold the mandibular incisors to their original position, thus ensuring maximum retention stability.

Lower Cuspid

First-order bend (in-out): **Thinner than regular**

Second-order bend (tip): **5°**

Third-order bend (torque): **–5°**

A thin bracket is necessary to compensate for the prominence of this tooth. The 5° tip is similar to that proposed throughout the literature. The –5° torque gives the lower cuspid a more labial version than in other prescriptions in order to articulate with the upper cuspid, as defined by this prescription. The torque is similar to that of the incisors. The cuspid tooth is thus positioned slightly lingual to the incisors (being at the corner of the arch). This supports the lower anterior dentition and should enhance postretention stability.

Lower First Bicuspid

First-order bend (in-out): **As thin as the lower cuspid**

Second-order bend (tip): **0°**

Third-order bend (torque): **–15°**

A thin bracket is required because of the similarity of this tooth to the cuspid. The 0° tip is again similar to that suggested by the literature. The –15° torque provides a slightly greater elevation of the lingual cusp than that suggested by Andrews (–17°) to provide a solid occlusion with the opposing dentition.

Lower Second Bicuspid

First-order bend (in-out): **Same as the lower first cuspid**

Second-order bend (tip): **0°**

Third-order bend (torque): **–20°**

All compensations for this tooth are made for the same reasons as for the lower first cuspid.

Lower Molars

First-order bend (in-out): **Mesially thin/distally thick (10″)**

Second-order bend (tip): **5°**

Third-order bend (torque): **–20°**

For the same reasons described for the maxillary molars, an overcorrection of the first-order compensation of 10° is needed to counteract the mesial rotation imposed on the molars by the elastic chains of sliding mechanotherapy. The –5° tip maximizes the lower molar resistance to mesial tipping from the sliding mechanics and offers a "tip-back" effect by placing the roots mesially, thus contributing to anchorage control during space closure. The –20° torque allows for good intercuspation of the lingual cusps without allowing unnecessary extrusion.

Control of Movement

13

*T*he control of tooth movement obtained with the triangular (Bioefficient) brackets is based on the introduction of a totally new component of bracket design: the side elbow extensions. These account for excellent control of tip and rotation, as well as reducing the anchorage needed because of less friction (Figures 86–103).

Bodily movement associated with space closure and detailed intercuspation is attained with sliding mechanotherapy provided by elastomeric chains and elastics.

Elastomeric chain modules (power chains, or C-chains) are used in sliding mechanotherapy primarily to close spaces. The elastic chain is hooked on the most posterior molar tooth that is banded and is then stretched and placed on every bracket of each tooth all the way around the arch to the most posterior molar tooth. The "pull" of the chain has two major side effects: mesial molar rotation and lingual "dumping" of all the teeth of the arch. These are counteracted with a distal "toe-in" bend in a rectangular stainless steel archwire in the molar region and an increased curve of Spee in the upper and a reverse curve in the lower wire. In all chains, the greatest force decay occurs during the first hour, and also, the greater the initial force, the greater the force decay.

One may easily correct the rotation of various teeth with the help of elastic chains, in addition to the full engagement of the rectangular NiTi superelastic wire in the bracket slots. No wire-tie should be placed on the tooth to be rotated, so that the movement created by the force vector of the elastic chain may "spin" the tooth freely around its axis (see Figures 100, 101). The other side of the chain is placed on a tooth that is wire-tied onto the rectangular superelastic wire, unless this also needs to rotate, but in the opposite direction.

Elastomeric chains should be changed every 6 to 8 weeks. If they are replaced any earlier, initial tipping occurs, but the tooth does not have time to "upright" (root movement) as the force of the chain dissipates, thus accentuating the tipping of teeth during space closure and not promoting the desired bodily tooth movement.

Elastics have been a valuable adjunct of any orthodontic treatment for many years. Their use, combined with good patient cooperation, provides the clinician with the ability to correct both anteroposterior and vertical discrepancies. They are used primarily with rectangular archwires. The introduction of the flexible rectangular NiTi wires allows the clinician to obtain immediate torque control from the onset of orthodontic mechanotherapy and thus use elastics from the beginning of treatment.

The following elastics are suggested for clinical use:

Class-I elastics extend within each arch (intra-arch elastics) and are primarily used to close spaces, as adjuncts to the elastomeric chains.

Class-II elastics extend from the lower molar teeth to the upper canines (interarch elastics). They are primarily used to cause anteroposterior tooth changes (i.e., aid in obtaining a Class-I cuspid relation from a Class-II relation). If the lower second molars are banded and included in the mechanotherapy, it is best to extend the elastic from the first molar to the cuspid tooth to avoid extrusion of the second molar and creation of an open bite anteriorly. If the lower second molars are not banded, it is best to extend the elastics from the second premolars to the upper canines (or even to the lateral incisors for a longer horizontal vector) if they are to be used for over 2 months of treatment. If elastics are to be used for 2 to 6 weeks only, then one may extend them from the lower first molars to the upper cuspid teeth. This treatment regimen minimizes the side effects from the use of elastics (i.e., extrusion of the lower posterior teeth and labial tipping of the lower anterior teeth, lowering of the anterior occlusal plane and the creation of a "gummy" smile). If any TMJ discomfort occurs, elastics should be discontinued, at least temporarily.

Class-III elastics are the exact opposite of Class-II elastics: They extend from the upper molars to the lower canines and are used in the treatment of Class-III cases. They promote extrusion of the upper posterior teeth and flaring of the upper anteriors, along with lingual tipping of the lower anteriors. The same principles discussed previously apply for Class-III elastics as well.

Triangle elastics aid in the improvement of Class-I cuspid intercuspation and increasing the overbite relation anteriorly by closing open bites in the range of 0.5–1.5 mm. They extend from the upper cuspid to the lower cuspid and first bicuspid teeth.

Box elastics have a box-shaped configuration and can be used in a variety of situations to promote tooth extrusion and improve intercuspation. Most commonly, they include the upper cuspid and lateral incisor to the lower first bicuspid and cuspid (Class-II vector) or to the lower cuspid and lateral incisor (Class-III vector). All bicuspid teeth on one side can be extruded as well.

Anterior elastics are used to improve the overbite relation of the incisor teeth. Open bites up to 2 mm may be corrected with these elastics. They may extend from the lower lateral incisors to the upper laterals or central incisor teeth, or from the lower canines to the upper laterals. Caution is advised.

Asymmetric elastics are usually Class-II on one side and Class-III on the other. They are used to correct dental asymmetries. If a significant dental midline deviation is present (2 mm or more), an anterior elastic from the upper lateral to the lower contralateral lateral incisor should also be used.

Finishing elastics are used at the end of treatment for final posterior set-tling. In Class-II cases, the elastic begins on the maxillary cuspid and continues to the mandibular first bicuspid, and in the same "up-and-down" fashion it finishes at the ballhook of the mandibular first molar band. In an open-bite or Class-III case, the elastic begins at the lower cuspid, continues to the maxillary cuspid (see later), and finishes at the maxillary molar.

The elastics are attached to ballhooks on the brackets or to K-hooks (heavy ligature wires with an extension). They should preferably be worn full time (24 hours/day) for maximum effect, although 12 hours/day wear may be indicated to minimize their side effects. They should be changed once or twice a day because the elastics fatigue rapidly (in contrast to the elastomeric chains, which last 3 to 5 weeks). The recommended sizes for the various elastics are *anteroposterior elastics,* light; *vertical elastics,* light or heavy; and *finishing elastics,* light.

During the finishing stages of treatment, a superelastic wire may be placed in the arch in which we want the teeth to extrude with finishing elastics while a stainless steel wire is placed in the opposing arch. Because the stainless steel is about eight times stiffer than the same-size superelastic wire, one observes ease of movement without sectioning of the archwires. This is especially useful in the postsurgical extrusion of the lower premolars after a mandibular advancement (the superelastic wire is placed in the lower arch and the stainless steel in the upper.) In addition, superelastic wires may aid in the final settling of individual teeth if the wire is simply placed in the overslot section of the upper bracket or the underslot area for a lower bracket. This area is rectangular in shape, and thus a square or rectangular superelastic wire may move a tooth (especially a premolar) toward the occlusal plane without the need for bracket repositioning or a second-order bend.

Part of the orthodontic wire armamentium has been coil springs. Originally, coil springs were made primarily of stainless steel. The use of NiTi alloys has resulted in the production of a new generation of superelastic coil springs that deliver a lower and more constant force during deactivation. The superelastic Sentalloy NiTi alloy coil spring has desirable springback and superelastic properties that are not possible with the stainless steel-type coil springs, and thus tooth movement can occur more quickly, efficiently, and comfortably. At body temperature, the springs exert a *constant* force of 150 g. Regardless of the length of the coil spring or whether it is activated 5 or 15 mm, the force remains constant at 150 g. The coil springs deliver a superior clinical performance and open new treatment possibilities. Because this force is activated at body temperature, it cannot be bench tested. The concept of using superelastic NiTi coils to move the molars distally has been demonstrated in the literature. An open coil may be compressed sequentially between the molar teeth or between the premolars for an effective, sequential space opening until a Class-I cuspid relation is achieved. Closed coils may sometimes be used for cuspid retraction instead of elastomeric chain modules in sliding mechanotherapy.

Applying the triangular brackets (Bioefficient) on the teeth is a very easy procedure (Figures 104–130).

Figure 86

The control during movement of the triangular brackets is similar to that of a surfer. The surfer can easily balance on calm water without opening his legs or arms. The moment big waves develop, the surfer opens his arms and legs wide for tip and rotation control. (Courtesy of Dr. Luiz Carlos de Mesquita Cabral.)

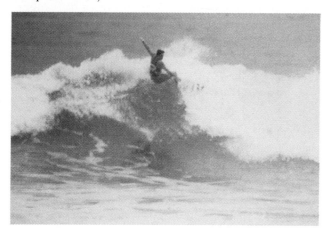

Figure 87

The bracket is the "surfer" and the wire the "calm" water. Note that the wire does not touch the elbows.

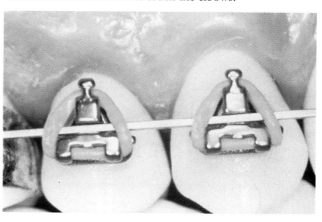

Figure 88

The biggest difference between the triangular bracket and any other twin design (full twin or uni) is the presence of the elbows. In other words, all other brackets are like the surfer without his arms. How can you surf without them? The elbows are the arms of the triangular bracket.

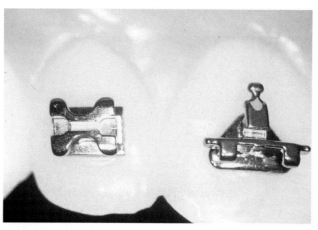

Figure 89

On movement, the elbows will touch the wire, and the intraslot distance then becomes X_1 to X_2 and the interslot distance, Y_1 to Y_2. In other words, the slot changes from single (X_1) to a wide twin (X_2)! On initial tipping of the tooth owing to tooth movement (as in space closure), the archwire contacts the elbows and thus the narrow single slot momentarily becomes a wide twin slot that results in root movement (because of the movement from the wide two-point contacts at the slot and the elbow) before any further crown movement takes place. Thus, the tooth "walks" back in a "zig-zag" manner. In other words, the new design becomes *a dual-slot bracket system when needed*. The interelbow distance is much smaller than the interslot distance and thus the same wire between the elbows becomes much stiffer, which results in better leveling and root parallelism before any further crown movement takes place. The tooth movement is continuous and controlled from crown to root to crown to root, and so forth.

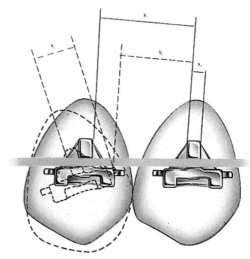

Figure 90

Imagine this lower arch as the sea. The "wave" is the wire and each bracket is a "surfer." The only tooth that is definitely tipped and needs uprighting is the canine. Note that the wire touches the elbows (X_2), or the "surfer" is using his arms to control the tip because of the "wave" of the wire. The canine bracket now has an X_2 slot (wide twin). All the others do not touch the elbows of the adjacent brackets, and thus the slots are X_1 (single type); in other words, why should the "surfer" use his arms if the "water" is calm, or the teeth are more-or-less straight?

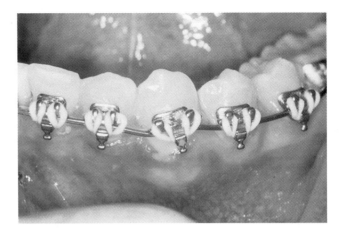

Figure 91

After 2 months, all slots are X_1 because now that the teeth are straight, the wire is straight, the "wave" is gone, the "surfer" does not have to use his "arms" (elbows), and the twin slot, X_2, is not needed and therefore is not present on any bracket. Movement is accomplished on X_2 (wide-twin slot) for maximum control, and when no movement is needed, the slot becomes X_1 (single type).

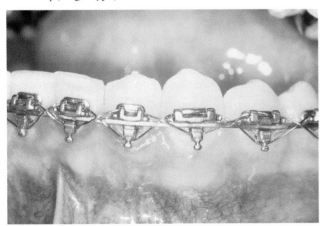

Figures 92–94

The triangular design allows for maximum interslot distance (Figure 92) for maximum wire flexibility during insertion and minimum interbracket (interelbow) distance for maximum control during movement (Figure 93).

Figure 92

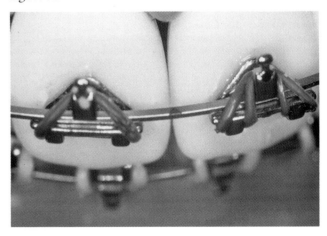

Figure 93

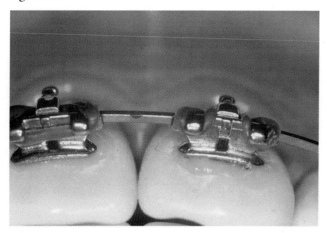

Figure 94

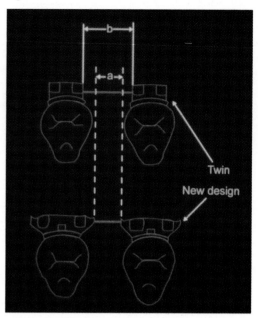

Rotational Control

Figures 95–97

Rotational control is achieved in a way similar to the way a car controls its speed on the race-track. Think of the bracket as a five-speed gearbox, except reversed. The first gear allows the car to go the fastest (the elastomeric modules are *over* the elbows-no friction) and the fifth gear (the elastomeric modules are behind the elbows—a lot of friction) the slowest (in fact, fifth gear is similar to the brakes of the car). First gear is shown on the right of Figures 95 and 96 and fifth on the left. First gear does not touch the wire with the elastomeric module, resulting in no friction (see Section II, Chapter 14) and therefore fast movement. In fifth gear, the module touches the wire (Figure 97), and therefore the "brakes" are applied and the bracket "car" stops.

Figure 95

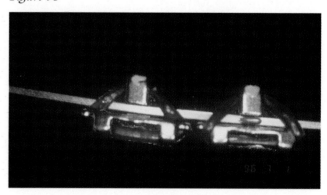

Figure 96

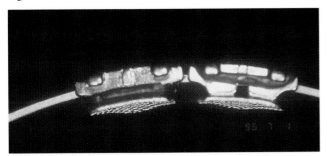

Figure 97

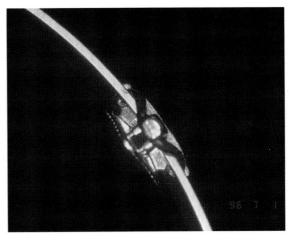

Figures 98, 99

The double-tie (right upper bracket) shown here is third gear of the system. When the elastomeric triangle module is behind one elbow only, this is second gear. When the double-tie is behind one elbow only, then it is fourth gear (left upper bracket). Remember, the friction (control) increases with the higher gear. Note, on Figure 99, the nice rotation effect achieved on the upper right central incisor from "fourth gear."

Figure 98

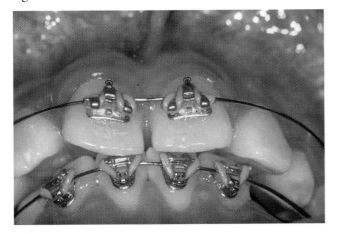

Figure 99

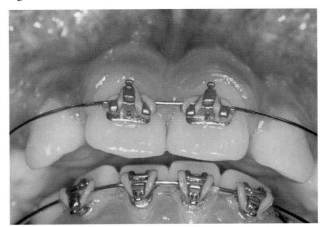

Figures 100, 101

Elastomeric chains may be attached in a number of ways onto the triangular wings of the bracket to produce a "spin" effect on specific teeth, such as the canine here. All the colored elastomeric chains appear capable of generating force levels compatible with physiologically sound tooth movement. Although changes in dimension were observed for the chains on storage in fluid media, the magnitude of such changes does not appear to be clinically relevant.

Figure 100

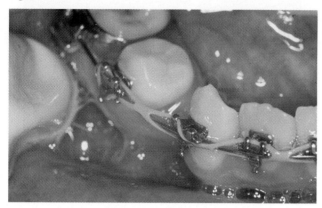

Figure 101

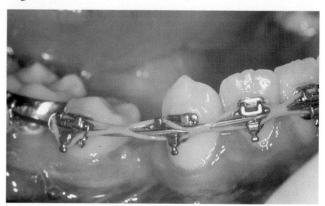

Anchorage Control

Figures 102, 103

Anchorage requirements in low-friction mechanics are much less than the conventional perception. The forces observed suggest that friction may be a significant influence on the amount of applied force required to move a tooth in the mouth. Hence, archwire and bracket selection may be an important consideration when posterior anchorage is critical. In most instances, to obtain a Class-I canine relationship, the canine tooth needs to move into the extraction space of the first premolar without loss of anchorage. All the clinician has to consider is the number of roots to be placed in opposition with each other in each unit. For example, if the posterior unit is composed of the first molar (three roots) and the second premolar (one root), and the anterior unit is the canine (one large root) and the incisor teeth (two roots), we have a total of four posterior roots against three anterior roots. This will cause both units to move into the extraction space, thus resulting in anchorage loss. When, conversely, individual canine retraction is used (one anterior root) and the posterior unit is composed of the second and first molars and the second premolar (a total of seven posterior roots), it is easily seen that the canine tooth will move posteriorly almost without any anchorage loss (i.e., mesial movement of the upper posterior teeth). Individual retraction of the premolars first is shown here. They will be followed by the canines.

Figure 102

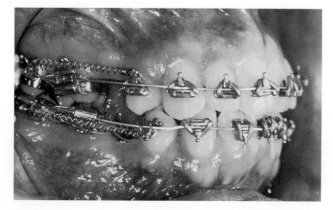

Figure 103

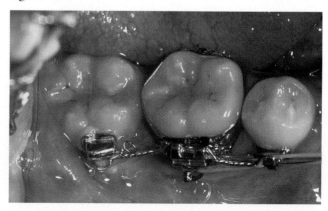

Figures 104–111

Direct bonding of triangular orthodontic brackets is a one-step process. The bracket heights are shown in Figure 105. The brackets of this prescription are diagonally shaped, with torque in the base. The base has an anatomically contoured triangular shape. The upper central incisor bracket is placed so that the middle of the tooth (FA point of Andrews) coincides with the slot of the bracket. If the distance of the bracket base to the incisal edge is X and that for the lower, Y, the brackets heights should be:

	\multicolumn{7}{c}{Tooth}						
	1	2	3	4	5	6	7
Upper	X	X − 0.5	X + 1	X	X	X − 0.5	X − 1
Lower	Y	Y	Y + 1	Y	Y	Y − 0.5	Y − 1

Note that the canine brackets must be a little higher to secure canine guidance. Note in Figure 106 that the brackets are all placed along the long axis of the teeth. Each bracket is custom-made for each tooth, because the angle between the vertical and horizontal members of the brackets differs for each tooth according to its individual long axis/incisal edge orientation (Figures 107, 108). The bands are bonded with a glass ionomer cement. With a glass ionomer cement, although band fitting and placement are still important for successful performance, decalcification is rare because of the fluoride-releasing property of the cement. Even when an oversize band loosens, the cement maintains its chemical bond to the enamel and forms a protective ring around the tooth. Although the minimum amount of fluoride release required to inhibit caries has not yet been determined, glass ionomer cements have been shown to leach fluoride ions directly into the enamel for at least 12 months. Only a few pliers are needed in the modern practice of orthodontics.

The *Howe* pliers: the clinician's "hand" in the mouth; mostly used to place the archwire in the bracket slots and to debond brackets. The Howe pliers can be used to manipulate the insertion of the "soft," cool-temperature wire in the bracket slots (Figure 107).

The *three-prong* pliers: used to bend larger size wires, such as the 0.030-inch round retainer wire and clasps.

The *hemostat:* used to place elastomeric modules, elastic chains, and ligature wires over the bracket wings.

The *wire cutter* pliers: used to cut wires outside of the mouth.

The *distal-end cutter* pliers: used to cut the archwire distal to the molar tube in the mouth.

The *band-sitter:* facilitates the smooth fit of the molar bands around these teeth.

The *band remover:* has a soft end, which contacts the tooth surface, and a metal end, which dislodges the band from its position.

The *cotton pliers/bracket-holding pliers:* used to place brackets onto the tooth surface.

The *3-mm periodontal probe:* aids in the accurate placement of the brackets onto the teeth.

The *bird-beak* pliers: used to bend stainless steel wires.

One of the most important design characteristics of the triangular bracket is its conformity to the premolar surface (Figures 110, 111). This is an extremely important adjunct to patient comfort and happiness. The bracket design conforms nicely to the gingival outline of the crowns of the teeth. This is especially useful for the bicuspids, where the brackets can now be placed as far gingivally as they need to be because the gingival portion of the brackets has a narrow, rounded end. The brackets have a low profile and blend well with the wire. The side elbows are hidden behind the elastomeric modules and are not visible after ligation. The peak of the triangle allows the bracket to be positioned next to the gingival contour of the tooth, thus avoiding occlusal interference and bracket failures. Other conventional bracket designs (square or with wings) do not provide the same conformity, and therefore bracket failures and hygiene problems would surface more readily.

Figure 104

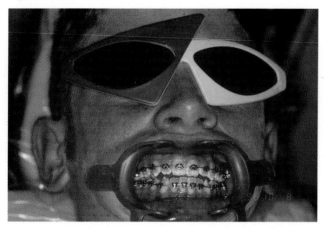

Figure 105

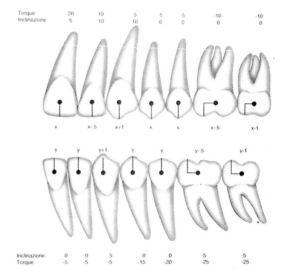

Figure 106

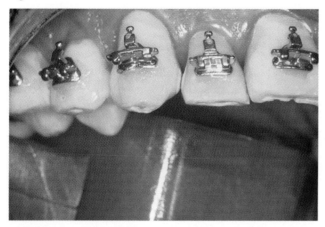

Figure 107

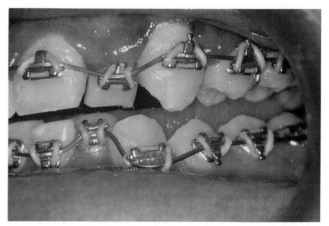

Figure 108

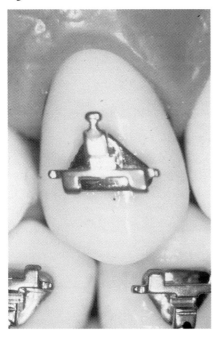

Figure 109

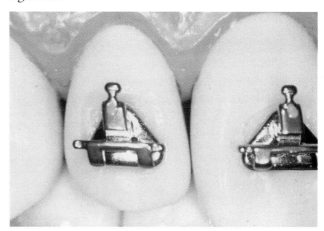

Figure 110

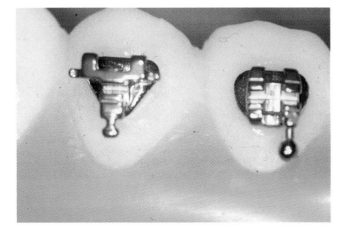

Figure 111

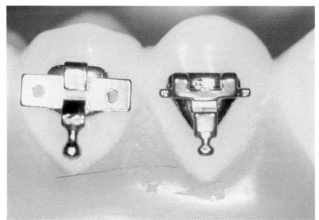

Preparing the tooth surface to receive the brackets involves etching for 15 seconds (Figure 112), rinsing and drying for 15 seconds (Figure 113), and applying the liquid of the adhesive system (Figure 114, 115). No pumicing is necessary as long as the patient maintains good oral hygiene.

Figure 112

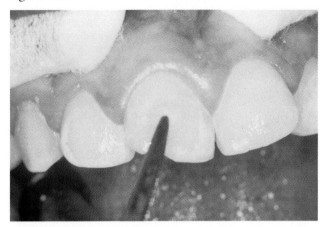

Figure 113

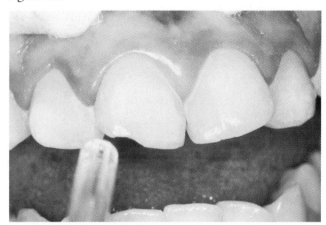

Figure 114

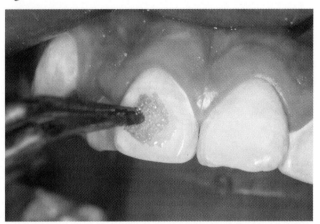

Figure 115

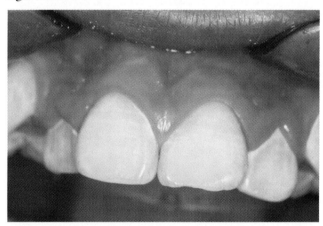

Figure 116

The liquid of the adhesive is applied on the bracket base before application of the paste.

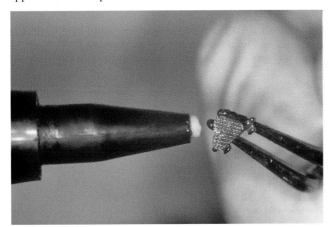

Figure 117

The paste covers a small portion of the middle of the bracket base.

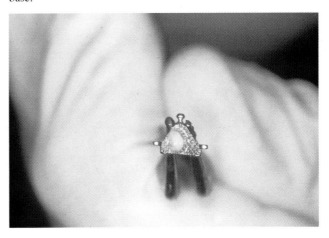

Figures 118–120

The triangular bracket (Bioefficient) design is extremely easy to place; all one has to do is aim the vertical member toward the center point of the curvature of the gingiva (soft tissue outline around the tooth). The vertical member of the bracket should be along the long axis of the tooth. The bracket is placed in the middle of the tooth with a small cotton pliers holder. The bracket should simultaneously be aligned with the long axis of the tooth. A periodontal probe may be used to measure the distance in millimeters from the incisal edge. For those clinicians using the bracket without the ball indicators, the vertical member may be aligned with the long axis of the tooth and check with the periodontal probe. The elbow side extensions also help with correct bracket orientation on the tooth surface because they point toward the mesial-distal sides of the crown. The incisal edge of the tooth (if normal in shape) should be parallel to the horizontal member of the bracket. Efficient ligation of elastomeric modules is very important because failure to do so may lead to significant additional chair time and staff frustration, along with patient discomfort. This bracket design makes ligation extremely easy and secure. One may use both the wings and the elbows.

Figure 118

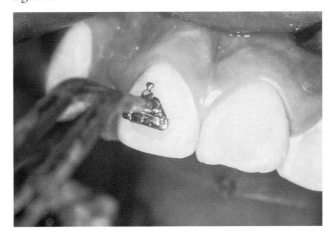

Figure 119

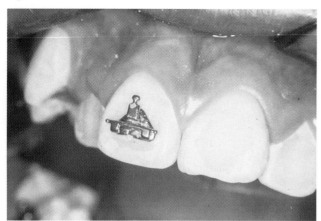

Figure 120

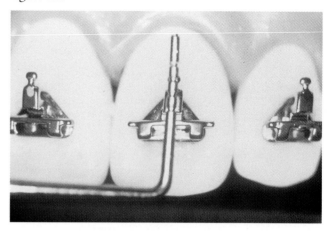

Figures 121, 122

The simultaneous positioning of the brackets based on the long axis of the tooth with the cotton roll-holding pliers is obvious. Thus, the lateral incisor is immediately positioned along the long axis of the tooth.

Figure 121

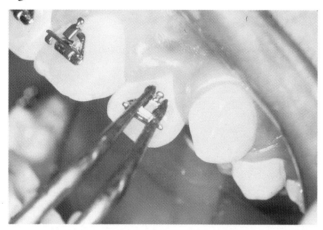

Figure 122

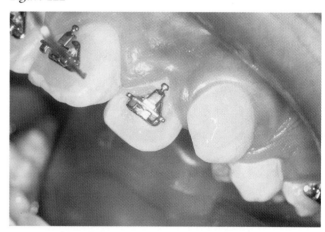

Figures 123, 124

The canine bracket is positioned so that its horizontal member is parallel to an imaginary flat incisal edge, as shown with the periodontal probe. This is because the soft tissue gum anatomy around the canine bracket may at times be misleading.

Figure 123

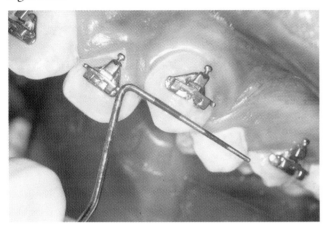

Figure 124

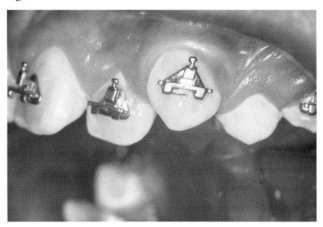

Figure 125

The lower incisor brackets are all placed at the same level from their incisal edge. They look like arrows pointing downward.

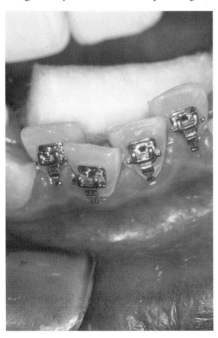

Figures 126–128

The triangular brackets are small and conform to the somewhat triangular shape of the teeth. Note the premolar region. The premolar brackets could easily be positioned more gingivally.

Figure 126

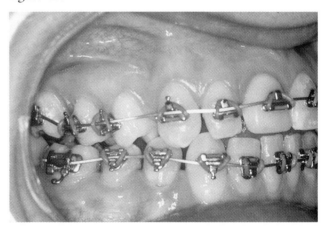

Figure 127

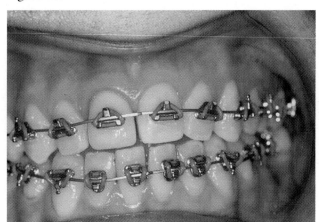

Figure 128

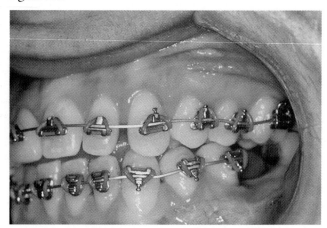

Figures 129, 130

The torque effect on the single-type slot can be quite significant. Shown here is the effect of a 15° buccal root torque that was placed on the upper left central incisor, resulting (in just 3 months) in a significant bulging of the root buccally.

Figure 129

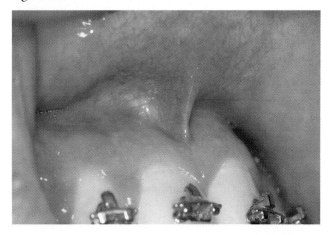

Figure 130

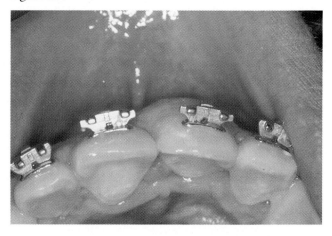

Friction: A Review

Michael R. LaFerla

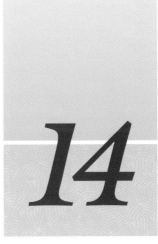

With the common use of preadjusted appliances, sliding mechanics is an important part of orthodontic treatment. For sliding mechanics to work, the resistance to movement commonly referred to as "friction" must be overcome.

Friction is independent of the surface area and depends on the characteristic surface being analyzed and the normal force being applied. The friction can be altered by modifying the characteristics of the surfaces in contact or the environment of the study as it is performed, or by varying the normal force as it is applied to the contacting surfaces.

The empirical laws of sliding friction state: (1) friction is proportional to the normal force, that is, the force pressing the two surfaces together; (2) friction is independent of the area of contact; and (3) friction depends on the state of smoothness of the surfaces in contact.

Materials are classified by a number called the coefficient of friction, which rates the relative amount of friction present in different materials. When determining the coefficient of friction, two coefficients must be distinguished: static and kinetic. The coefficient of static friction depends primarily on the nature of the surfaces in contact, with rough surfaces having larger coefficients and smooth surfaces having small coefficients. The coefficient of static friction is the ratio of the maximum possible frictional force parallel to the surface of contact, which acts to prevent two bodies in contact and at rest from sliding past each other. The coefficient of static friction always has a higher numerical value than that of kinetic friction, because of the need for the bodies being measured to overcome inertia.

The coefficient of kinetic friction is the ratio of the frictional force parallel to the surface of contact, which opposes the motion of one body that is sliding past another. The value for the coefficient of kinetic friction remains approximately dependent on the speed.

Proffit believes that frictional resistance to sliding in orthodontic appliances is multifactorial, with microscopic irregularities, commonly referred to as asperities, as a contributing factor. These elevated areas carry all the load between two surfaces and may cause plastic deformation with enough force. Thus, the true contact area is determined by the applied load. Large asperities may cause interlocking of surfaces or digging into the opposing surface. Proffit states that a "stick–slip" phenomenon may occur at a low sliding speed. The wire may stick until enough force is present to make it slip past, and then the wire may stick again with the cycle starting over.

Andreasen and Quevado (1970) were the first to perform an in-depth friction study evaluating the frictional forces in the 0.022 × 0.028-inch edgewise bracket system. Numerous round and rectangular stainless steel wires, three bracket widths, four bracket–wire angulations, and wet/dry state were studied, with 72 possible combinations analyzed. Results indicated increased frictional resistance to sliding with an increase in wire size and increase in angulation. The bracket width and wet/dry conditions were found to be insignificant.

This first study led to numerous studies on the role of friction in orthodontics. Many variables are involved in the total frictional resistance to sliding of an archwire through the slot of an orthodontic bracket. Some of the variables include surface roughness, wire material, wire size, wire shape, ligation material, presence of lubrication, bracket material, bracket width, bracket slot size, and bracket–wire angulation.

Surface Roughness

Several studies have attempted to determine the relation between surface roughness and the coefficient of friction. Laser spectroscopy and scanning electron microscopy have been used to determine surface roughness of the various wires available. Roughness was ranked from stainless steel (smoothest), to beta-titanium (intermediate), to nickel-titanium (roughest). The coefficient of friction had only slightly positive correlations to surface roughness except for beta-titanium, whose correlations were inconsistent and normally ranked with the highest coefficient of friction even though its surface measured smoother than nickel-titanium.

Wire Material

Previous studies have consistently ranked the various wires available for use in orthodontics based on coefficient of friction and frictional resistance to sliding. In these studies, wires of the same dimensions were compared under experimental conditions with no bracket offsets. The rankings consistently demonstrated stainless steel lowest, nickel-titanium intermediate, and beta-titanium highest.

Wire Size

Previous studies have consistently agreed that as the wire dimension increases, so does the frictional resistance to sliding. As the wire size increases, it leaves less slop in the bracket slot and increases the wire stiffness, which results in higher frictional resistance to sliding.

Wire Shape

The wire shape also has an impact on the frictional resistance to sliding. Round wires tend to have lower frictional resistance to sliding than square and rectangular wires of the same material and size under the same experimental conditions. Lower frictional resistance to sliding is expected to be found with round wires because they do not bind the bracket corners as much during sliding movements. With square and rectangular wires, the binding or notching effect between the wire and bracket corners would produce higher frictional resistance to sliding. Increase in wire stiffness of similar-sized round, square, or rectangular wires also creates the same effect.

Ligation Material

The type of ligature and force applied has a significant influence on wire engagement, which in turn affects the frictional resistance to sliding. Teflon-coated ligatures produce the least frictional resistance to sliding. The stainless steel ligatures vary significantly in the force produced when ligating. The operator controls the amount of force applied when tying the stainless steel and Teflon ligatures, which results in high variability when using these two methods. The instrument (e.g., hemostat, Mathieu pliers) used can also have an affect on the force level produced when ligating with stainless steel and Teflon.

The elastic ligatures consistently produce high friction, although the resulting friction is less than that with a tightly tied stainless steel ligature. The high variability of tying ligatures makes the use of elastic ligatures the most consistent and reproducible.

Lubrication

Lubrication from saliva has been implicated as a factor that increases frictional resistance to sliding in some studies and decreases frictional resistance to sliding in other studies. The variability in its role may be explained by saliva having varying effects on different wire materials. The role of saliva has yet to be well defined, but overall it seems to be of minor importance. Furthermore, because saliva is not easily controlled in patients, it tends to be more of a biologic situation that a clinician simply cannot regulate.

Bracket Material

Bracket material has become a very popular test subject with the addition of esthetic brackets. The research shows a significant difference between stainless steel and ceramic brackets. Ceramic brackets, although a greater esthetic value to the patient, has shown higher coefficients of friction and frictional resistances to sliding than stainless steel brackets. The addition of plastic brackets reinforced with metal inserts has brought about a new area for friction research. No friction study to date has analyzed these new brackets.

Bracket Width

Bracket width correlation to frictional resistance to sliding has been controversial. Some studies suggest little correlation between frictional resistance to sliding and bracket width, whereas others suggest the opposite. The studies that have shown an increase in frictional resistance to sliding values have suggested that the use of elastomeric ligatures stretched over the wider brackets causes a tighter ligation of the wire into the bracket, resulting in increased friction. These studies did not repeat the tests using stainless steel or Teflon ligatures to prove their hypothesis. Results from studies on bracket width are inconclusive.

Bracket Slot Size

Bracket slot size has been shown to be an insignificant component of frictional resistance to sliding because the wire size associated with the bracket slot determines the frictional resistance to sliding. When comparable wire sizes are tested in either the 0.018 or 0.022-inch slot size, the frictional resistance to sliding differences are statistically insignificant.

Bracket–Wire Angulation

One of the largest frictional resistance to sliding determinants seems to be the angulation of interface between the bracket slot and the archwire. Numerous studies have concluded that frictional forces increase as the angulation between the bracket slot and archwire increase. The different wire types react differently; stainless steel, being the stiffest wire, has the most rapid frictional resistance to sliding increase with angular increase. Nickel-titanium has also been shown to undergo an increase in frictional resistance to sliding as the angulation increases, but it is significantly lower compared with that of stainless steel. Beta-titanium has an increase in frictional resistance to sliding as well, but the increase appears to lie in between that of nickel-titanium and stainless steel.

Conclusions

The study discussed throughout this chapter was initiated to determine the effect of ion-implantation on frictional resistance to sliding for nickel-titanium and beta-titanium archwires. Another objective was to determine the frictional resistance to sliding of plastic brackets with metal inserts, and to compare these values to ceramic and stainless steel brackets. All the information obtained in this study is clinically relevant and may be directly applied in patient treatment.

1. Ion implantation lowers frictional resistance to sliding in the Bioforce archwire.
2. Ion implantation of TMA arch wire alone does not reduce frictional resistance to sliding.
3. Plastic brackets with metal inserts have lower frictional resistance to sliding than ceramic brackets.

4. Plastic brackets with metal inserts have comparable frictional resistance to sliding with some stainless steel brackets.

5. Bracket design plays a large role in frictional resistance to sliding, as seen with triangular brackets, which have shoulders to hold the ligature away from the archwire.

6. Elastic ligatures that are tightly stretched on large brackets may be a key determinant in frictional resistance to sliding.

Additional comments extracted from study:

1. Differences were also seen among the stainless steel brackets, with triangular brackets having significantly lowest mean frictional forces—by 87% compared with all the other brackets in the study (Figures 131, 132).

2. In analyzing the data, bracket design seemed to make a large difference in frictional resistance to sliding. The triangular bracket showed extremely low readings regardless of the wire being tested.

The effects of low friction can be seen in figures 133–200.

Figure 131

The first friction study on triangular brackets was conducted to the University of Santiago in Spain (European study). The researchers concluded that friction with the brackets can be up to 10 times less than that with conventional brackets. (Courtesy of the University of Santiago, Compostella, Spain.)

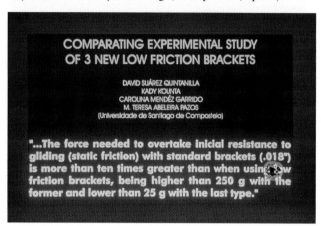

Figure 132

The European study showed that the friction with the triangular brackets (Viazis) can be up to 10 times lower regardless of the wire being used. (Courtesy of the University of Santiago, Compostella, Spain.)

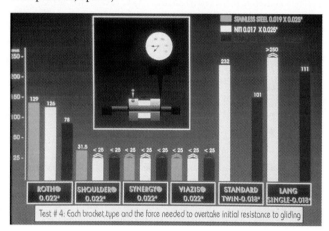

Figure 133

The new, very–low-friction triangular brackets. Note the small size and conformity to the tooth surfaces.

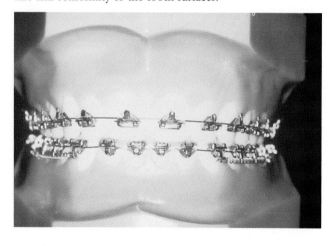

Sliding Space Closure

Figure 134

A triangular bracket being retracted distally as it slides on the wire. Imagine the tooth as an ice skater, skating on smooth ice (triangular brackets) versus rough ice (some conventional square brackets). The skater's legs (roots of the teeth) glide faster and easier on smooth versus rough ice, with less effort from the legs (less force on the teeth).

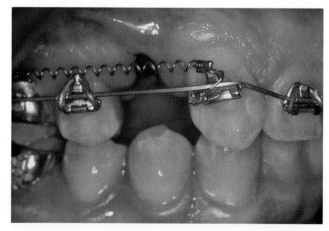

Figure 135

Based on the European study, the triangular brackets (Viazis) were almost twice as fast under simulated, in vitro conditions compared with some conventional brackets. (Courtesy of the University of Santiago, Compostella, Spain.)

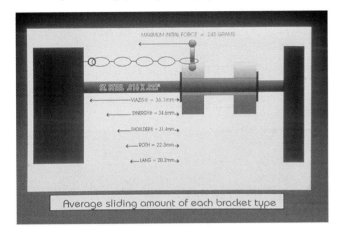

Figure 136

The second independent university study that confirmed the efficiency of the triangular brackets was conducted at the University of Southern California (Los Angeles, California). (Courtesy of Dr. Michael LaFerla.)

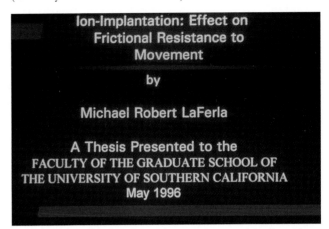

Figures 137, 138

Various contemporary wires and brackets were tested. (Courtesy of Dr. Michael LaFerla.)

Figure 137

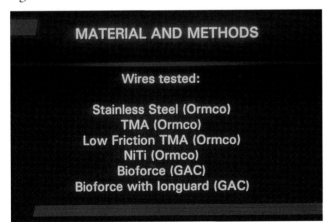

Figure 138

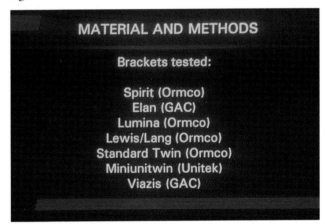

Figure 139

The results showed that regardless of the wire being tested, the Viazis triangular brackets (Bioefficient) can produce up to 10 times lower frictional forces compared with various contemporary conventional brackets. The Viazis triangular brackets had the significantly lowest mean frictional forces, by 87% compared with all the other brackets in the study. (Courtesy of Dr. Michael LaFerla.)

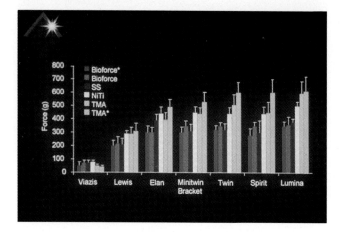

Figure 140

The ion implantation treatment of the Bioforce wire produced an 11% reduction of friction in the brackets. Therefore, the combination of triangular brackets (Viazis) with an ion-treated wire would provide the most frictionless environment available today. To conclude, reduction in friction results in fast and easy movements with a treatment time of approximately 1 year for a lot of patients, regardless of whether an extraction or nonextraction modality is used. (Courtesy of Dr. Michael LaFerla.)

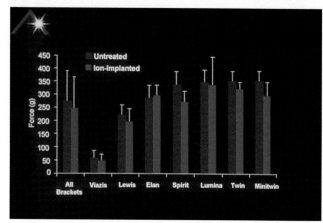

Figure 141

Initial activation of teeth with a 20 × 20 Bioforce Ionguard wire in a 0.022-inch slot triangular bracket. Note the extreme position of the teeth.

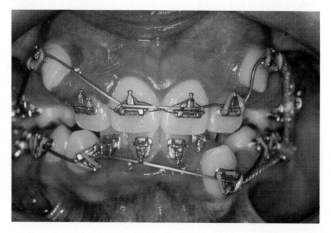

Figure 142

Same patient 2 months later. Note the dramatic movement of the canines in a very short period of time. The patient was very comfortable.

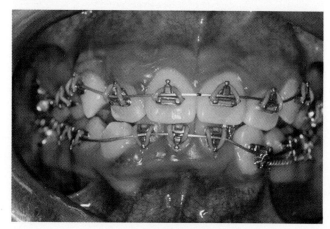

Section II: *Treatment*

Figure 143

Same patient 8 months into treatment with the finishing 19 × 25 stainless steel wires in place.

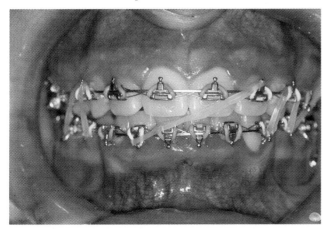

Figure 144

Same patient 10 months into treatment. The patient will soon finish. The same case would have taken at least twice as long with conventional twin brackets and stainless steel wires.

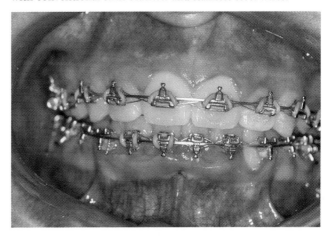

Figures 145, 146

This patient had the upper right first molar and the upper left first premolar extracted. The triangular brackets were used with the superelastic wire. Five months into treatment, the extraction spaces are almost completely closed and the teeth have been brought into alignment. This would have taken well over a year with conventional mechanotherapy.

Figure 145

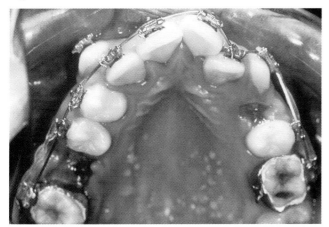

Figure 146

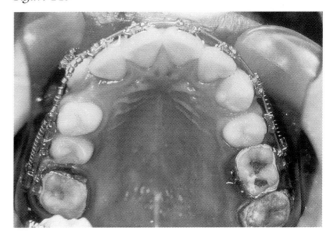

Figures 147, 148

This patient's orthodontic treatment with triangular brackets was completed in less than a year.

Figure 147

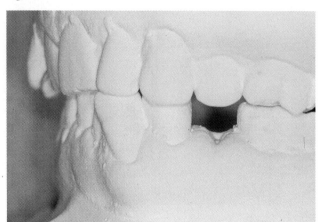

Figure 148

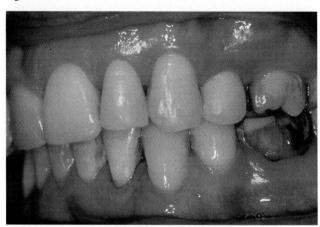

Alignment
Leveling   *Part 1*
Space Closure

Finishing   *Part 2*

In the past, we had alignment *of the* crowns: *today we can have* alignment *of the* crowns *and the* roots!

Figure 149

In the past, the orthodontist would spend an average of 6 months aligning teeth, another 6 months leveling, 6 months closing spaces, and 6 months finishing. In other words, the treatment would be divided into four stages. Today, treatment can be divided into two parts. In part 1, alignment, leveling, and space closure can now be accomplished simultaneously. In particular, alignment of the crowns and roots can take place from the beginning of treatment. Part 2 (finishing) is emphasized because the clinician spends half of his or her time detailing the occlusion.

This patient was going to have a lower incisor removed. No bracket was placed on that tooth. Brackets were placed on the rest of the teeth to "energize" the cells (osteoclasts and osteoblasts) so the moment the tooth is extracted the adjacent teeth can move right into the extraction site. The intentional extraction of a lower incisor can enable the orthodonist to produce enhanced functional occlusal and cosmetic results with minimal orthodontic manipulation. If the Bolton analysis shows a lower anterior excess, the extraction of a lower incisor might have a positive effect. Enamel removal can be distributed among 10 maxillary interproximal surfaces (the mesial surfaces of both canines and proximal surfaces of the 4 incisors) to compensate for lower incisor extraction and reduce any excess overjet at the end of treatment. The proximal enamel is usually thickest on the mesial surfaces of the canines and the distal surfaces of the central incisors, whereas the mesial surfaces of the lateral incisors may have only 0.5 mm of enamel. If the interproximal surface is indiscriminately flattened, the interproximal contact will be lengthened gingivally, further reducing the space for the gingival

Figure 149 (continued)

papilla. Extruding the lower incisors to maintain occlusal contact in centric occlusion is advised. If the maxillary anterior tooth size excess is managed successfully, one can usually still achieve a canine-protected occlusion. In some cases, it is impossible to compensate adequately for the tooth size imbalance, so it may not be possible to achieve a canine rise. In these cases, group function may be produced orthodontically and by equilibration to eliminate cross-arch balancing interferences.

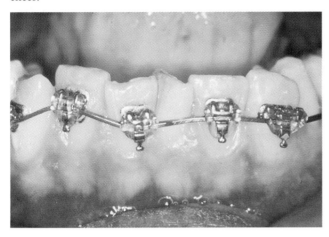

Figure 150

Two months into treatment.

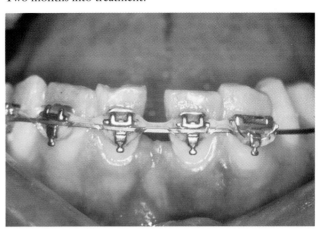

Figure 151

Three months into treatment.

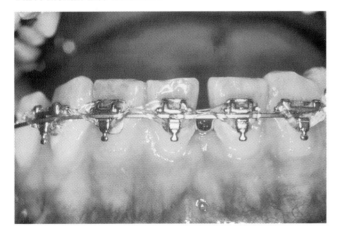

Figure 152

After 4 months of treatment, the space is closed.

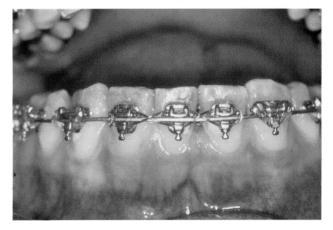

Figure 153

Overall view of the interior region of the same patient before the extraction.

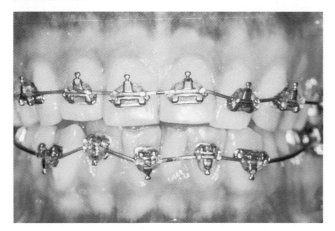

Figure 154

After the extraction. Note the fresh extraction site, and the already significant movement of teeth into the site.

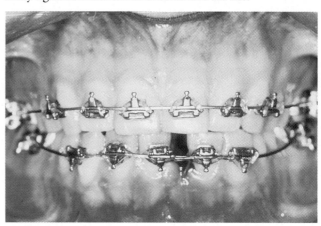

Figure 155

Two months into treatment.

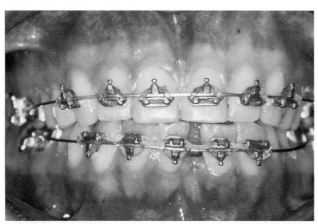

Figure 156

Three months into treatment.

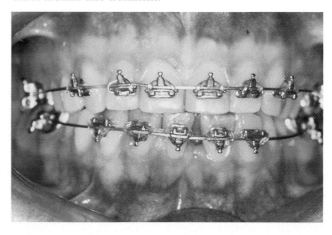

Section II: *Treatment*

Figure 157

Four months into treatment, with the space closed.

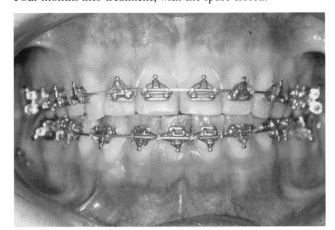

Figure 158

Eight months into treatment. Note the beautiful intercuspation of the teeth. It took as much time to close the space as to bring the case to completion. The case was completed in less than a year, but most of the treatment time was spent detailing the occlusion.

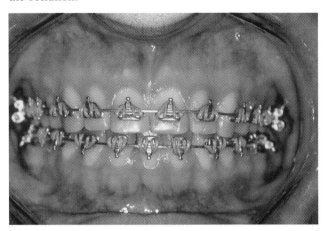

Figures 159, 160

Checking canine guidance on the right with working and balancing clearance.

Figure 159

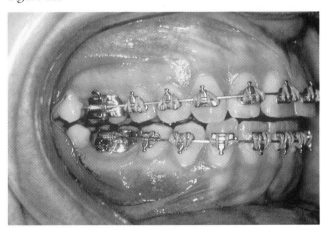

Figure 160

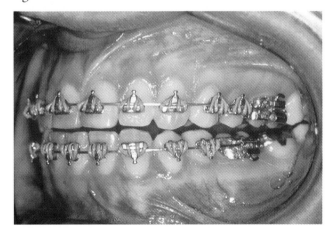

Checking canine guidance on the left with working and balancing clearance.

Figure 161

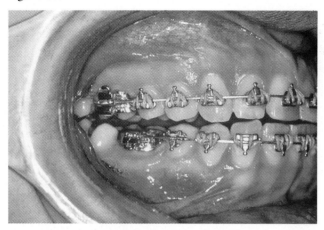

Figure 162

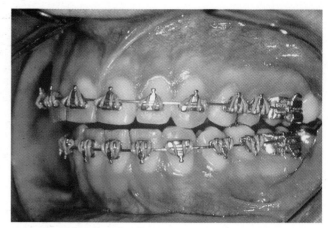

Figures 163, 164

Patient's final occlusion before removal of the brackets.

Figure 163

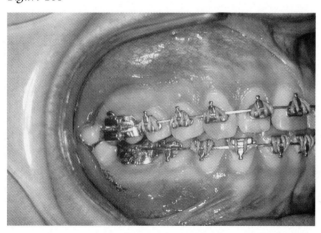

Figure 164

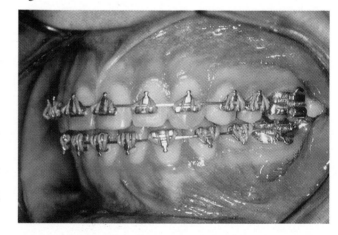

Root Parallelism

Figure 165

The roots should be parallel, like telephone poles. This cephalometric tracing confirms that borderline cases such as this one benefit greatly from lower incisor extraction therapy.

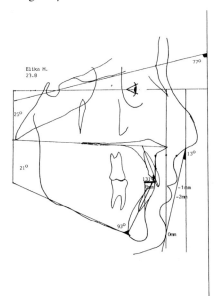

Figures 166, 167

This adult patient's chief complaint was the crowded lower incisors. Mandibular incisor extraction therapy is indicated in carefully selected cases, especially where space requirements and facial esthetics do not call for greater dental movements.

Figure 166

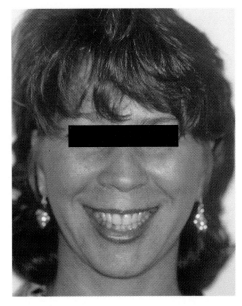

Figure 167

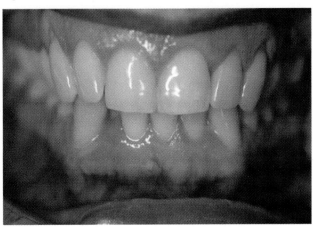

After 6 months of lower incisor extraction therapy. The patient was amazed at the speed and comfort of treatment.

Figure 168

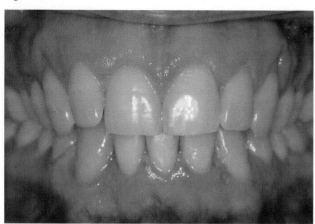

Figure 169

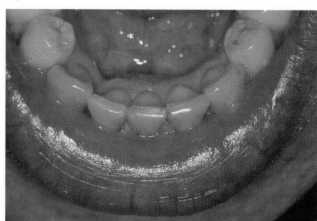

Figures 170–172

Close-up views demonstrating proper root alignment, parallelism, and an esthetically pleasing lower smile contour. The patient did not wish to have any therapy of the upper arch.

Figure 170

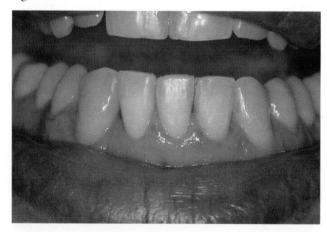

Figure 172

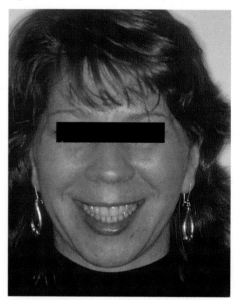

Figure 171

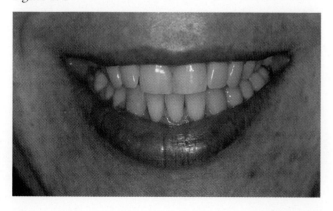

A case from the past...

Figure 173

This case was treated with the mechanics of the past. The upper first premolars and the lower second premolars were extracted to bring the canines into a Class-I relation. Today this case would have been treated by nonextraction.

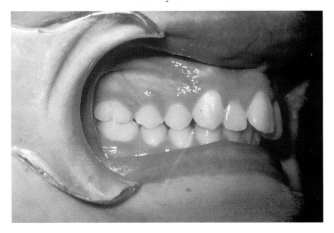

6 months

Figure 174

It took 6 months to go through the regular sequence of stainless steel archwires of 0.012, 0.014, 0.016, 16 × 16, and finally 16 × 22, as shown here in the 0.018-inch bracket slot. Space closure is finally initiated.

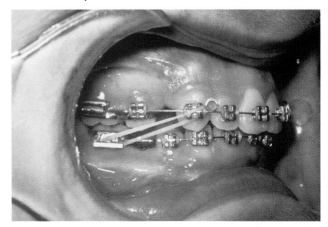

18 months

Figure 175

It took a whole year from the initiation of space closure finally to close the spaces.

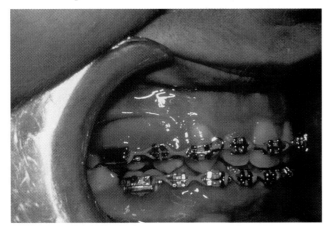

24 months

Figure 176

It took approximately 2 years to bring this case to completion. This case could have been treated in much less time with contemporary mechanotherapy of superelastic wires in triangular brackets, because the space closure could have been initiated from the beginning of treatment.

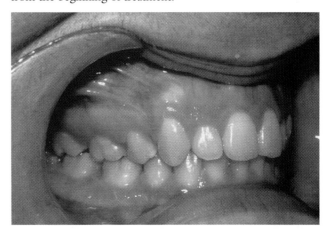

Figures 177, 178

This case was treated with contemporary mechanotherapy. Because of the bimaxillary protrusion and dental crowding, the upper and lower first premolars were extracted.

Figure 177

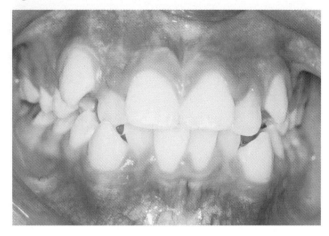

Figure 178

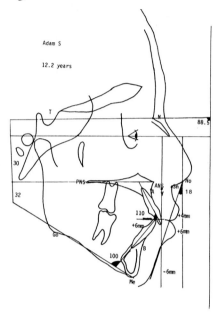

Figure 179

Patient shown here with triangular brackets (0.022-inch slot) in place at the first appointment. The superelastic wires (20 × 20) and coil springs will bring the teeth into position. The large-size wires will allow for control of the slot during the movement.

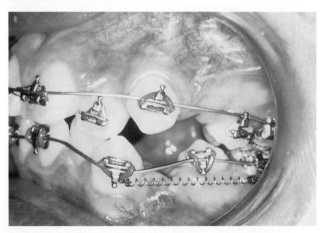

Figure 180

Two months into treatment. Note the significant retraction of the canines and the leveling that has already taken place.

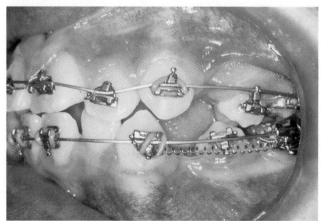

Figure 181

Three months into treatment.

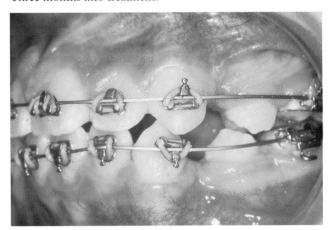

Figure 182

Four months into treatment.

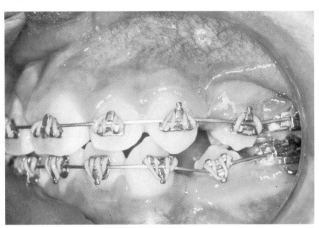

Figures 183, 184

Six months into treatment, with stainless steel wires (19×25) in place and space closure on its way to completion. Note the beautiful root structure, and parallelism on the panoramic radiograph. Fast movement with light forces does not result in root resorption.

Figure 183

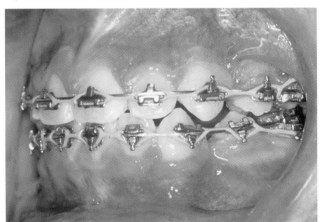

Figure 184

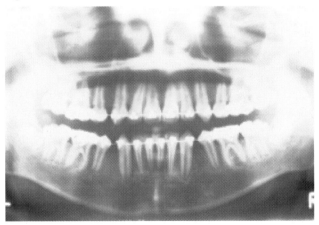

Figure 185

Ten months into treatment.

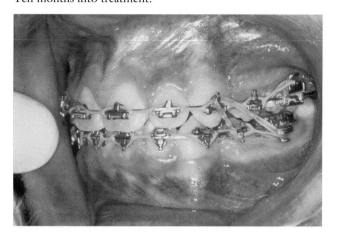

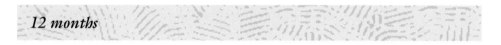

12 months

Figures 186, 187

Twelve months into treatment, the patient is almost ready to have the appliances removed. Compared with the case shown in Figures 173 to 176, the treatment time has been halved.

Figure 186

Figure 187

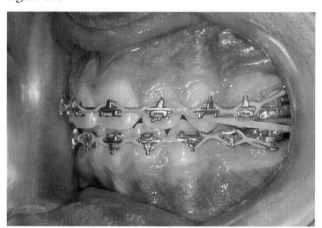 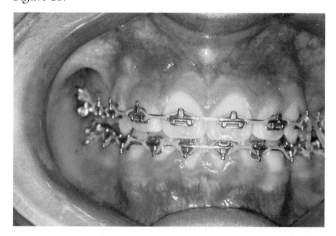

Figure 188

A case from the past and a case from the present are compared in the next sequence of photographs (Figures 188–200). Both cases have had the upper first premolars and the lower second premolars extracted. The case treated with the old mechanics (stainless steel wires, small wire sizes, square brackets) still has the canines and lower incisors well out of alignment.

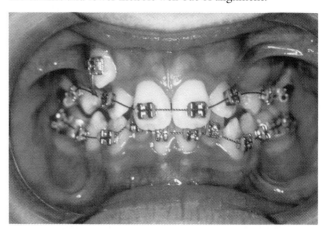

2 months

Figures 189, 190

The case treated with the new mechanics (superelastic wires, large wire size, triangular brackets) demonstrates rapid tooth movement and alignment of canines and lower incisors teeth within the first 2 months.

Figure 189

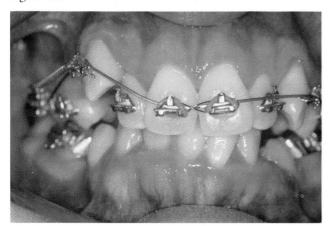

Figure 190

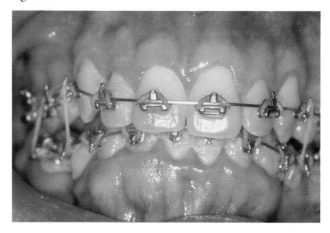

Figure 191

Eight months into treatment, and the canines still have not been brought into alignment with the old mechanics (note the box loop on the upper left canine used with stainless steel mechanics to reduce wire stiffness).

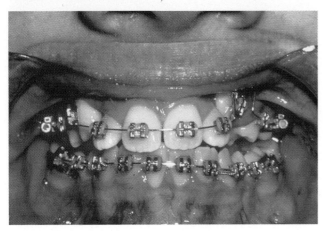

Figures 192, 193

Contemporary mechanotherapy with the new wires and brackets has, by the eighth month of treatment, brought all anterior teeth into beautiful alignment.

Figure 192

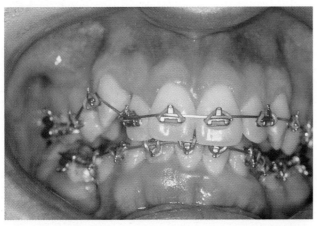

Figure 193

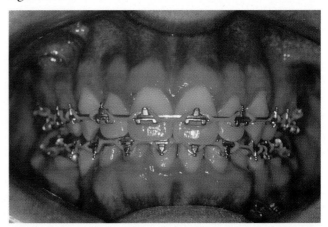

Figures 194–197

The patient treated with contemporary mechanics shown from a buccal view, from the beginning through the eighth month of treatment. Note the significant anterior as well as posterior tooth movement with the same archwire as it slides in the low-friction environment of the triangular brackets.

Figure 194

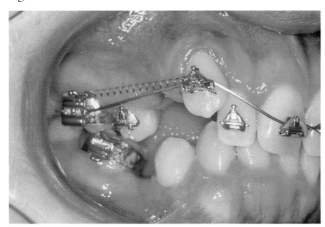

Figure 195

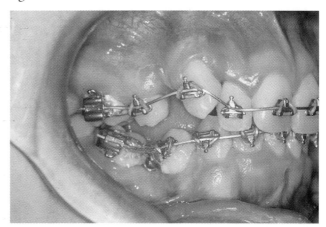

Figure 196

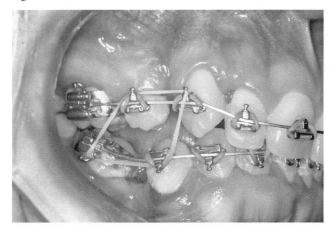

Figure 197

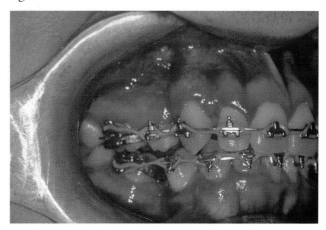

Figure 198

It took 18 months of treatment with the old mechanics to finally close all the spaces.

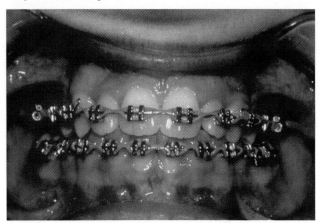

Figures 199, 200

It took just 9 months with the new mechanics to close the spaces—half the time of the previous case.

Figure 199

Figure 200

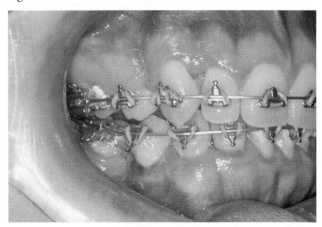

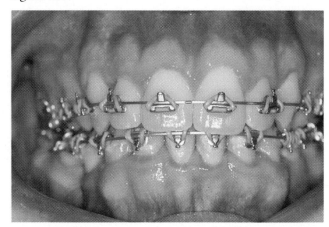

Nonextraction Therapy

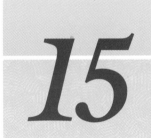

15

Contemporary orthodontic mechanotherapy leads to treatment results that are based on the six keys to normal occlusion: (1) a Class-I molar relation (or today, Class-II or III as long as the cuspid is in Class-I); (2) crown angulation (tip)—the gingival portion of the crown of teeth is distal to the incisal portion in most individuals; (3) crown inclination (torque)—anterior crowns have an anterior inclination, whereas posterior crowns have a lingual inclination; (4) absence of rotations; (5) absence of spaces; and (6) the plane of occlusion should be flat or have a slight curve of Spee (Figures 201–419).

Tooth recontouring is defined as air-rotor stripping of the posterior teeth (mesial of first molar to distal of cuspid) with a fine diamond burr with plenty of water irrigation, and as interproximal reduction with a disc of the incisor teeth and mesials of the canines. This method resolves mild (1–3 mm) to moderate (4–7 mm) crowding by reducing enamel where the greatest amount of enamel is present—distal to the canines. As much as 0.5 to 1 mm is removed from each tooth, thus allowing for about 3 mm of space in each quadrant. This space is used to alleviate anterior crowding. Bulky bicuspid teeth are ideal for such a procedure.

The clinical recommendations for tooth recontouring are to use abundant water cooling and carefully grind with a diamond instrument. One must always prepare a smooth and self-cleansing surface.

The mesiodistal enamel reduction (stripping) procedure is becoming increasingly used as an alternative to tooth extraction, particularly in nongrowing patients. Using a correct enamel reduction technique, up to several millimeters of crowding can usually be resolved by stripping. Even in cases where there is no evident tooth size discrepancy between the maxillary and mandibular teeth, stripping may be advantageous in several situations. If there is slight crowding (less than approximately 4 mm), stripping may eliminate the need for extraction of permanent teeth. A more stable result is established by broadening the contact area and eliminating small contact points with potential for slippage and subsequent rotations of teeth. Often, areas of interproximal gingival recession may be improved with mesiodistal enamel reduction. To establish a more favorable overbite and overjet relation for the anterior teeth, use the stripping technique to improve the anterior function in the mutually protected occlusion.

Several indicators have been presented as to the amount of enamel that may be removed, including 0.5 mm in each tooth contact, the Peck and Peck ratio (mesiodistal length divided by buccolingual width), and so forth. More enamel can be removed in "triangular" teeth than in teeth with more parallel interproximal sufaces. It may not be possible to remove any enamel at all in some teeth. The amount of enamel removed by mesiodistal enamel reduction depends on crown morphology.

Stripping is, of course, not restricted to use on anterior teeth. In several instances, reduction in the width of enamel or fillings is of value in the premolar and molar regions as well. This is particularly useful in adult cases.

Results of a recent study indicate that the roughness produced by recontouring does not predispose to caries. Remineralization appears after 9 months. These findings substantiate those of other studies that found no increased susceptibility to caries or periodontal disease after stripping. Therefore, a sealant would only delay the remineralization that occurred between 6 and 9 months. However, topical application of fluoride after recontouring should be encouraged.

In the tooth recontouring technique, a NiTi coil spring is placed first between the first molar and the second bicuspid. After 2 weeks, a 2-mm space has been created. The mesial of the molar and the distal of the second bicuspid are recontoured with a fine diamond burr; 0.25 mm of enamel is removed from each side. The next step is to place the coil spring between the first and second bicuspid and so on. In this manner, space is created sequentially from the posterior to the anterior region.

In addition to tooth recontouring, expansion therapy contributes to nonextraction. Expansion appliances may be used to correct unilateral or bilateral posterior crossbites involving several teeth when the discrepancy between the maxillary and mandibular first molar and bicuspid widths is 4 mm or more. The applied pressure acts as an orthopedic force that opens the mid-palatal suture. The amount of sutural opening is reported to be equal to or less than one half the amount of dental arch expansion. The increase in the intermolar width can be as much as 10 mm, with a mean increase of 6 mm. During the retention period there is uprighting of the buccal segments; therefore, one can appreciate the need for overcorrection of the dental arches. Because the mid-palatal suture may ossify as early as 15 years and as late as 27 years of age, the optimal period of sutural expansion is between 8 and 15 years of age. Treatment with the rapid palatal expander presents good stability for upper intercanine width, upper and lower intermolar widths, and incisor irregularity.

The patient's guardian is instructed to turn the screw once a day (each turn equals approximately 0.025 mm) for a month for a total of 7 mm of expansion. The appliance is then sealed with acrylic (care should be taken to avoid contact with soft tissue) for another month, at which time a maxillary Hawley retainer is given for 6 to 9 months of full-time wear if the patient is in the mixed dentition stage. In the permanent dentition, the superelastic wire may be placed after the expansion as long as overcorrection has taken place. After expansion, the lingual cusps of the maxillary posterior teeth should be at the level of the buccal cusps of their mandibular counterparts. No transpalatal arch is used. The buccal segments will show a strong tendency toward relapse, but not beyond the normal buccolingual relation.

Where the mandibular posterior teeth seem to be lingually inclined as one looks at the dental casts, a lower expansion screw appliance is used to upright these teeth over basal bone and at the same time alleviate any anterior crowding. The screw is turned once a week for up to 6 months.

Andy . . . The first male patient treated with the triangular brackets

Total Treatment Time 16 months

Figure 201

Andy was the first male patient treated with the triangular brackets. His displeasing smile took away from his otherwise balanced facial characteristics.

Figure 202

After just 16 months of treatment, he was proudly displaying his new smile.

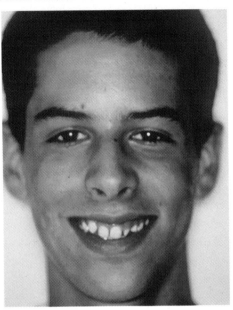

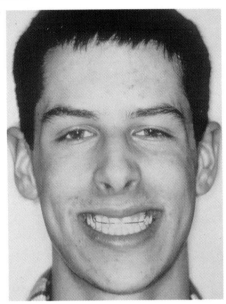

. . . and today

Figure 203

Today he is a young man with a beautiful smile, on his way to success.

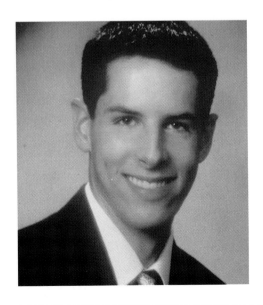

Figures 204, 205

Andy presented with a facial and profile appearance within normal limits.

Figure 204

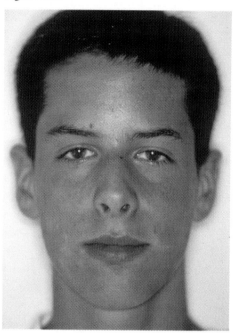

Figure 205

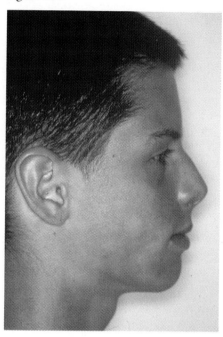

Figures 206, 207

His chief complaint was the awkward appearance of his smile. This was due to his missing upper right lateral incisor, the peg upper left lateral incisor, his canted occlusal plane, his deep bite, and his gummy smile.

Figure 206

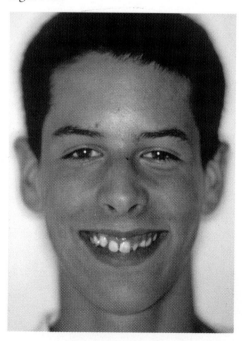

Figure 207

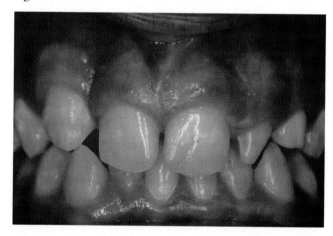

Figure 208

The missing upper right lateral incisor resulted in mesial drift of the upper right permanent canine. The upper left permanent canine was impacted because the primary tooth was still in place. The treatment plan was to open up space for an upper right lateral incisor prosthesis, build up the peg laterally, and bring the impacted canine into position in the arch.

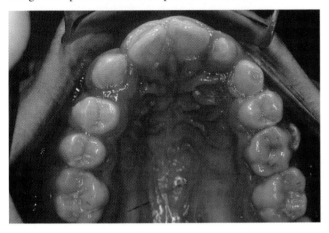

Figure 209

The lower arch had minor crowding that would be resolved with simple alignment of the teeth.

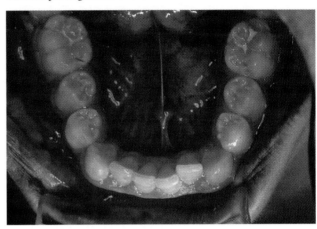

Figure 210

Upper occlusal view with the prototype triangular brackets in place.

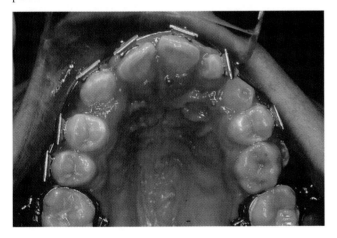

Figure 211

Within 6 months, the teeth were aligned.

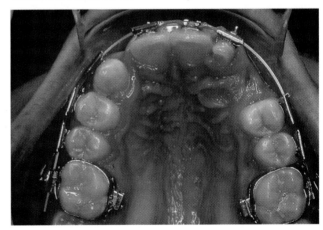

Figure 212

The impacted canine was uncovered 9 months into treatment because it did not show any signs of eruption on its own during the previous 6 months.

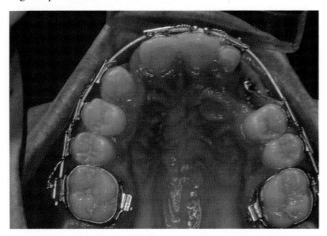

Figure 213

A little over a year into treatment, the upper arch is ready for the finishing details.

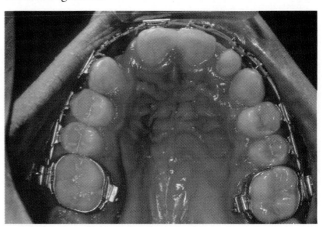

Figure 214

Right buccal view before treatment.

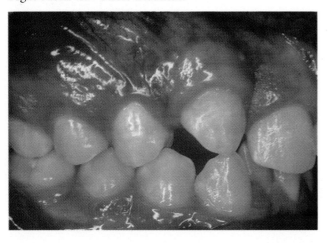

Figure 215

A year into treatment, the upper right lateral incisor space has been opened. Note the prototype of the triangular brackets.

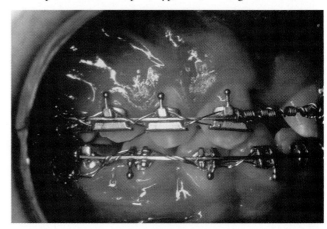

Figure 216

Fourteen months into treatment.

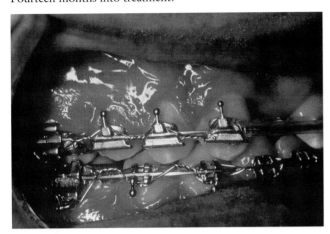

Figure 217

Fifteen months into treatment.

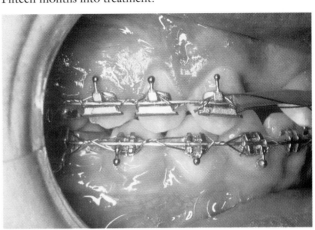

Figure 218

Sixteen months into treatment, the brackets were removed.

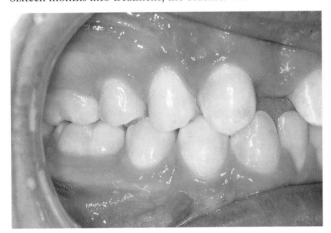

Figure 219

Left buccal view before treatment. Note the primary canine and the erupting second premolar.

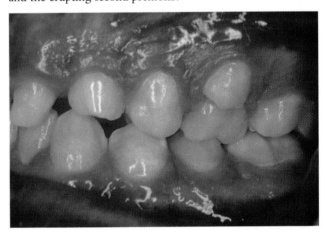

Figure 220

The impacted canine is uncovered and attached to the fixed appliances.

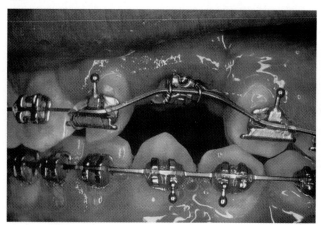

Figure 221

At the end of treatment, after 16 months of therapy.

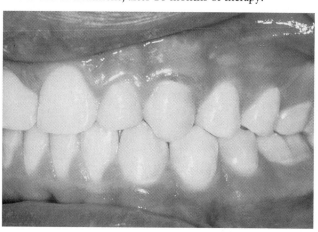

Figures 222, 223

Before and after views of the anterior dentition. Note the midline correction, the uprighting of the upper arch, the leveling of the occlusal plane, and the nice intercuspation of the canines.

Figure 222

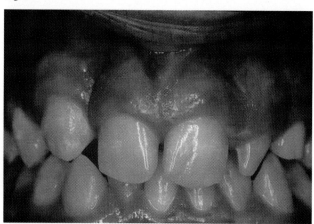

Figure 223

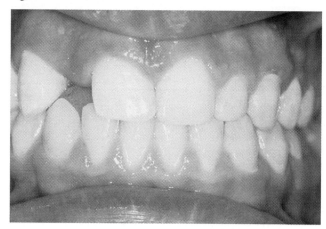

Figures 224, 225

Before and after cephalometric radiographs. Note the proper incisor inclinations after treatment.

Figure 224

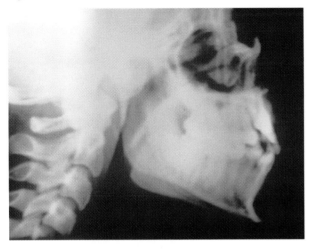

Figure 225

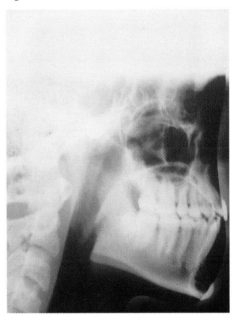

Figures 226, 227

Before and after profile views.

Figure 226

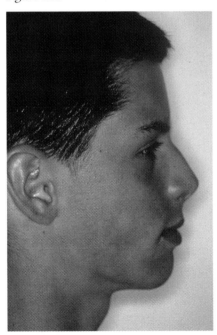

Figure 227

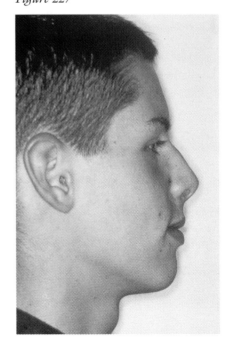

Andy's smile before, after, and with the retainer in place. Andy was going to have a prosthesis (bridge or implant) later.

Figure 228

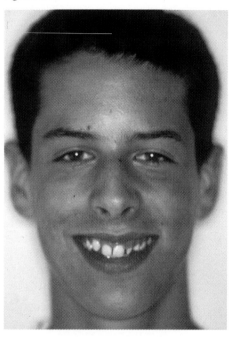

Figure 229

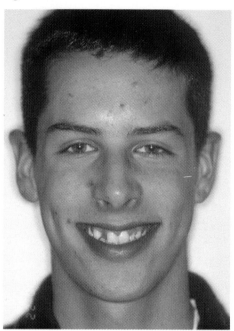

Figure 230

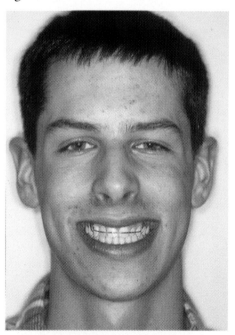

Figure 231

A young man's smile has changed forever.

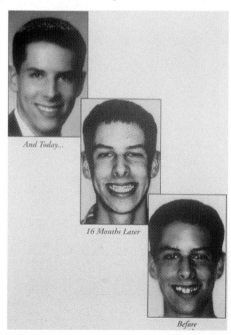

Figure 232

This patient's chief complaint was her narrow smile and crowded teeth.

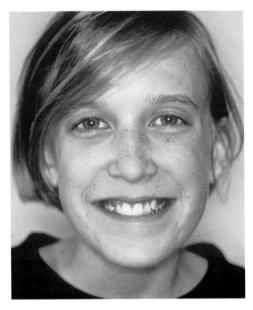

Figure 233

Kelly 14 months later, with a beautiful smile.

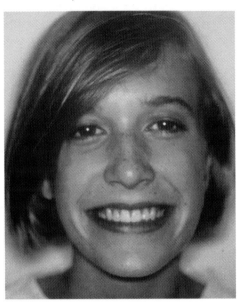

...and today

Figure 234

Kelly's beautiful smile today.

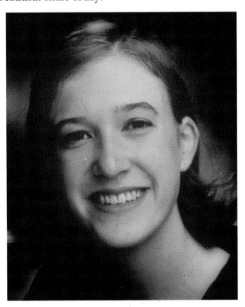

Figure 235

Anterior view before treatment. Note the left posterior cross-bite and the severe crowding in the upper arch.

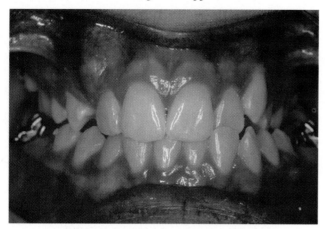

Figure 236

Anterior view after treatment. The therapy was nonextraction with expansion of the upper arch followed by upper and lower fixed appliances using just the superelastic wires.

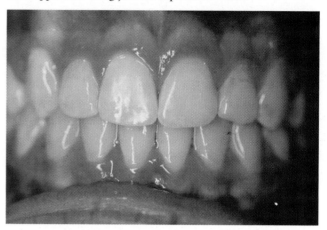

Figure 237

Upper occlusal view before treatment. Note again the severe crowding in the upper right canine area and the narrow arch.

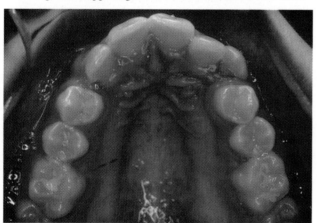

Figure 238

Upper occusal view after treatment. Note the beautiful, broad arch that resulted from sutural expansion and fixed appliance therapy in just a little over a year.

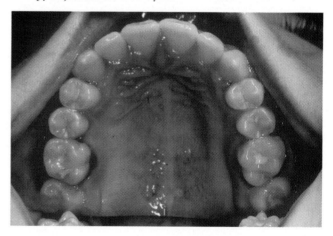

Section II: *Treatment*

Figure 239

Lower occusal view before treatment. Note the lingually inclined lower premolars.

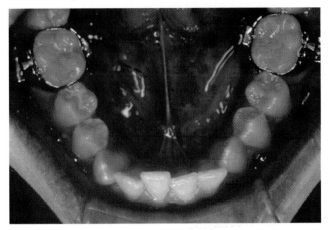

Figure 240

Lower occlusal view after treatment. The lower premolars were uprighted over basal bone with the broad superelastic wires. The lower arch now complements the broad upper arch.

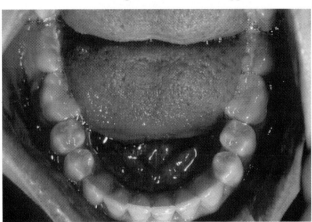

Figure 241

Patient's facial view before treatment.

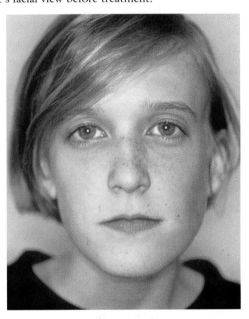

Figure 242

Patient's facial view after treatment.

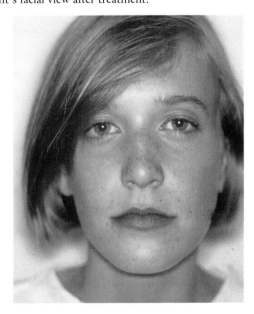

Figure 243

Patient's profile view before treatment.

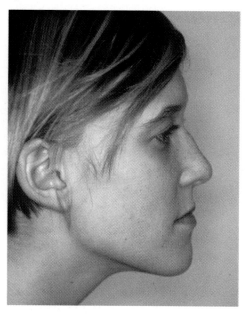

Figure 244

Patient's profile view after treatment.

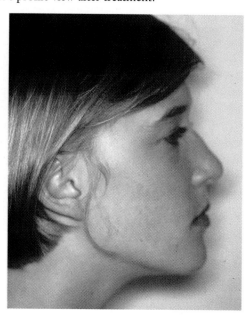

Figure 245

Patient's smile view before treatment.

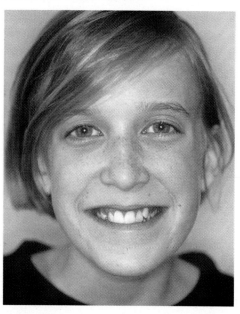

Figure 246

Patient's smile view after treatment.

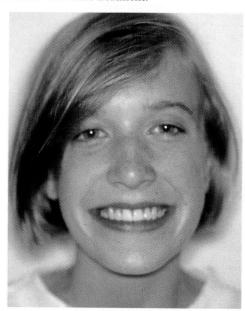

Section II: *Treatment*

Figure 247

Kelly's smile has changed forever.

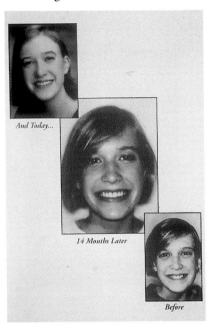

And Today...

14 Months Later

Before

Figure 248

The patient's facial view demonstrates a primarily dental problem. (Courtesy of Drs. Janson, Martins, Henriques, de Freitas, Pinzan, and de Almeida of the University of São Paulo, Bauru Dental School, Brazil.)

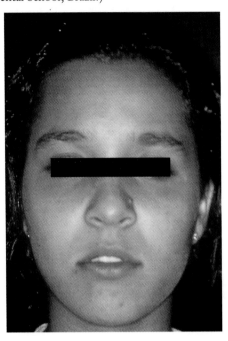

Figures 249, 250

This young patient's smile and profile views confirm a primarily dental problem. (Courtesy of Drs. Janson, Martins, Henriques, de Freitas, Pinzan, and de Almeida of the University of São Paulo, Bauru Dental School, Brazil.)

Figure 249

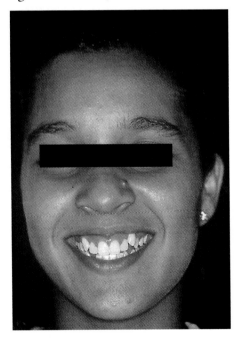

Figure 250

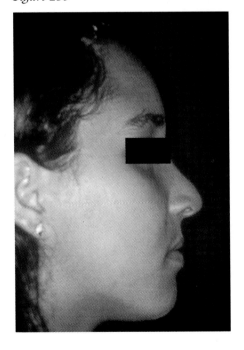

Figures 251–253

Patient's right anterior and left buccal views before treatment. Note the malformed upper right first molar, the crossbite tendency, and the blocked-out canines. (Courtesy of Drs. Janson, Martins, Henriques, de Freitas, Pinzan, and de Almeida of the University of São Paulo, Bauru Dental School, Brazil.)

Figure 251

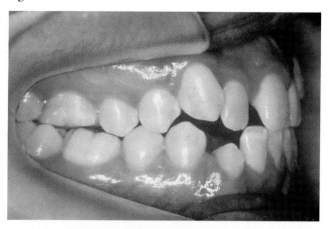

Figure 252

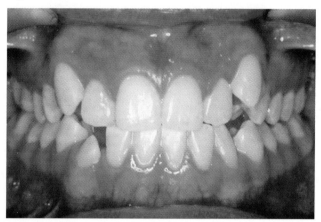

Figure 253

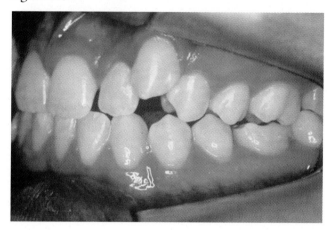

Figures 254, 255

The patient's anterior view before maxillary sutural expansion and after 1 month of expansion. Note the significant midline diastema, indicating good sutural opening. (Courtesy of Drs. Janson, Martins, Henriques, de Freitas, Pinzan, and de Almeida of the University of São Paulo, Bauru Dental School, Brazil.)

Figure 254

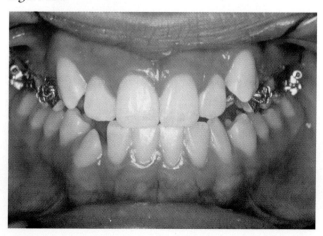

Figure 255

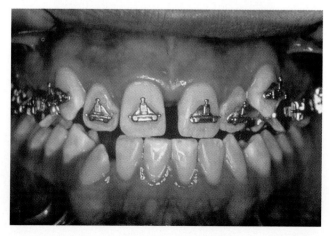

Figures 256–258

The triangular brackets were placed 2 months into treatment and after the expansion. Note the inverted "V" or double ties and the activation of the wire as it flows from bracket to bracket. (Courtesy of Drs. Janson, Martins, Henriques, de Freitas, Pinzan, and de Almeida of the University of São Paulo, Bauru Dental School, Brazil.)

Figure 256

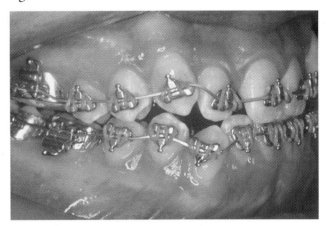

Figure 257

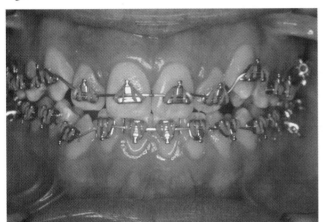

Figure 258

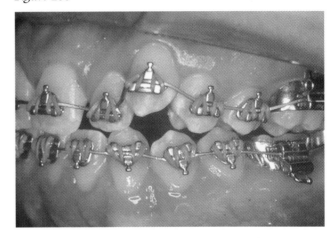

Figures 259–261

Two months later, note the significant leveling that has taken place in both arches. The superelastic wire is holding the correction very well. (Courtesy of Drs. Janson, Martins, Henriques, de Freitas, Pinzan, and de Almeida of the University of São Paulo, Bauru Dental School, Brazil.)

Figure 259

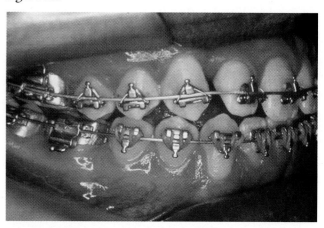

Figure 260

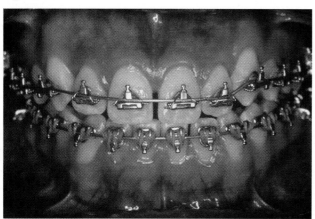

Figure 261

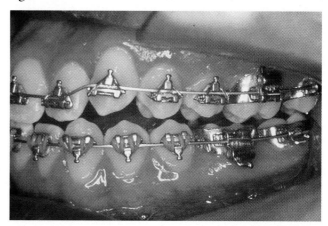

Figures 262–264

Two months later, the arches are completely level. Elastomeric chains are closing in the remaining spaces. Note the midline asymmetry. (Courtesy of Drs. Janson, Martins, Henriques, de Freitas, Pinzan, and de Almeida of the University of São Paulo, Bauru Dental School, Brazil.)

Figure 262

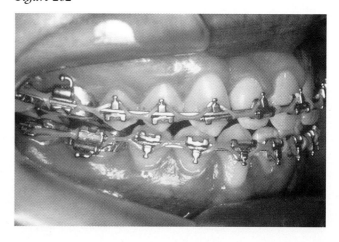

Section II: *Treatment*

Figure 263

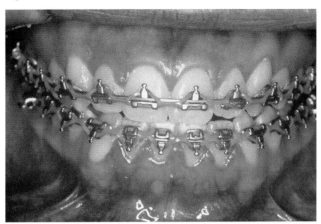

Figure 264

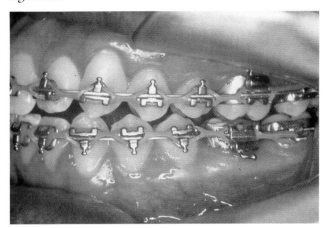

Figures 265–267

One month later, asymmetric elastics were added to correct the midline discrepancy. (Courtesy of Drs. Janson, Martins, Henriques, de Freitas, Pinzan, and de Almeida of the University of São Paulo, Bauru Dental School, Brazil.)

Figure 265

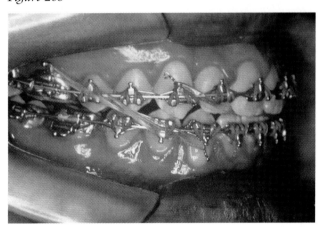

Figure 266

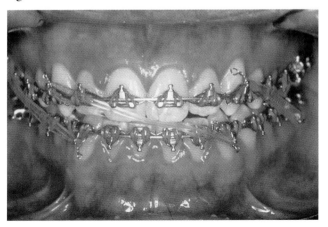

Figure 267

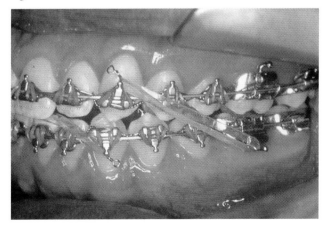

Figures 268–270

Two months later, the midline asymmetry is corrected. Note the overslot activation of the upper right first premolar. This activation eliminates the need for a second-order bend because the overslot area is rectangular in shape and can accommodate the wire nicely. (Courtesy of Drs. Janson, Martins, Henriques, de Freitas, Pinzan, and de Almeida of the University of São Paulo, Bauru Dental School, Brazil.)

Figure 268

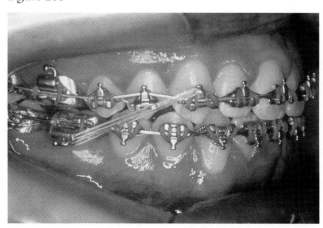

Figure 269

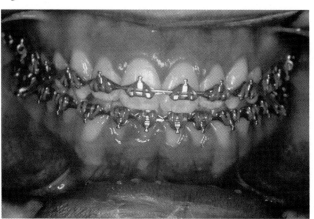

Figure 270

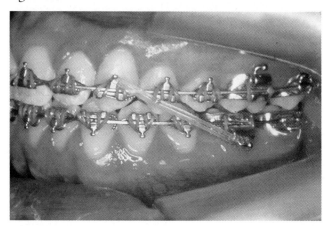

Figures 271–273

The patient got her brackets off after 14 months of treatment. Note the beautiful intercuspation of the teeth, the midlines, and canine positions. (Courtesy of Drs. Janson, Martins, Henriques, de Freitas, Pinzan, and de Almeida of the University of São Paulo, Bauru Dental School, Brazil.)

Figure 271

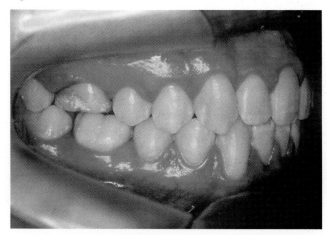

Figure 272

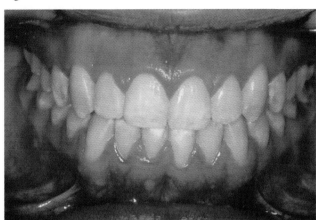

Figure 273

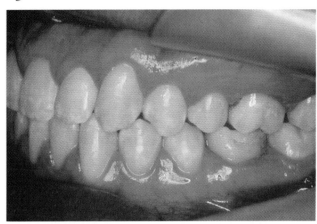

Figures 274, 275

The patient in protrusive and canine guidance demonstrating excellent occusal relation. (Courtesy of Drs. Janson, Martins, Henriques, de Freitas, Pinzan, and de Almeida of the University of São Paulo, Bauru Dental School, Brazil.)

Figure 274

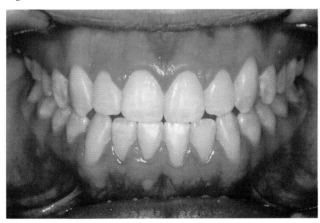

Figure 275

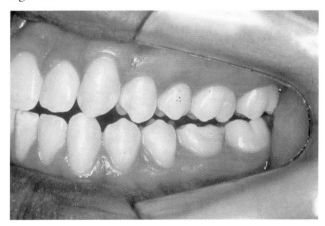

Facial, smile, and profile views after treatment. (Courtesy of Drs. Janson, Martins, Henriques, de Freitas, Pinzan, and de Almeida of the University of São Paulo, Bauru Dental School, Brazil.)

Figure 276

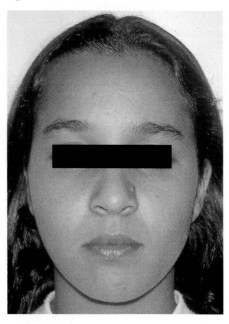

Figure 277

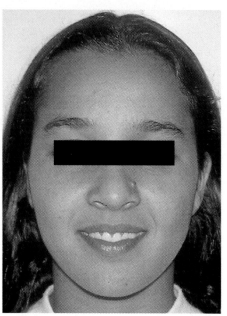

Figure 278

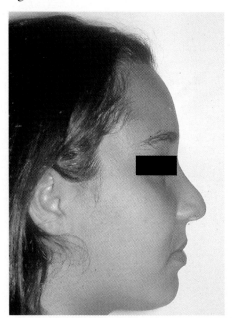

Figure 279

The cephalometric radiograph demonstrates excellent tooth positions and inclinations. (Courtesy of Drs. Janson, Martins, Henriques, de Freitas, Pinzan, and de Almeida of the University of São Paulo, Bauru Dental School, Brazil.)

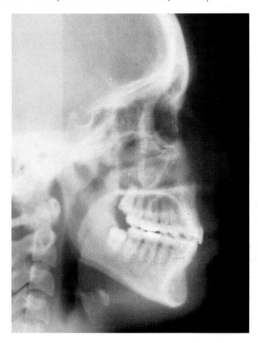

Figures 280, 281

The patient's panoramic radiographs before and after treatment. Note the beautiful root parallelism that was achieved. There is complete absence of any root resorption because the treatment was completed in a relatively short period of time, consistent with most cases treated with contemporary triangular bracket mechanics. (Courtesy of Drs. Janson, Martins, Henriques, de Freitas, Pinzan, and de Almeida of the University of São Paulo, Bauru Dental School, Brazil.)

Figure 280

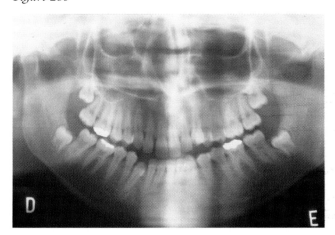

Figure 281

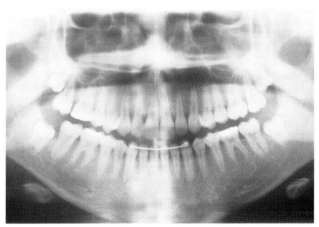

Figures 282–284

This boy's facial, profile, and smile views demonstrate a deep bite. (Courtesy of Drs. Janson, Martins, Henriques, de Freitas, Pinzan, and de Almeida of the University of São Paulo, Bauru Dental School, Brazil.)

Figure 282

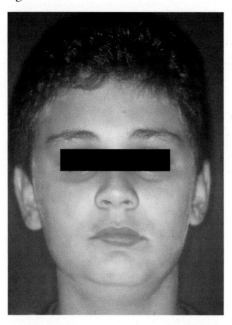

Figure 283

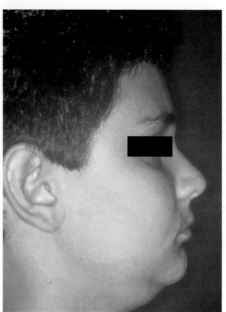

Figure 284

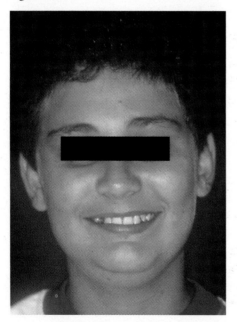

Figures 285–287

The right buccal anterior and left buccal views of the dentition demonstrate lack of adequate space for the canine teeth, midline discrepancy, and moderate overbite. (Courtesy of Drs. Janson, Martins, Henriques, de Freitas, Pinzan, and de Almeida of the University of São Paulo, Bauru Dental School, Brazil.)

Figure 285

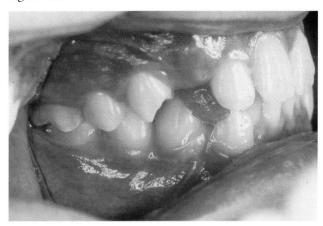

Figure 286

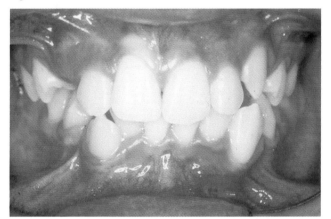

Figure 287

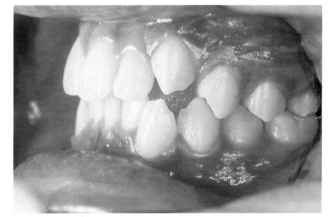

Figures 288–290

Upper and lower triangular brackets with a superelastic wire were placed at the first appointment. Note the significant wire activation. Contemporary mechanotherapy allows for complete manipulation of the wire in any direction without any discomfort for the patient, as long as the wire has been properly cooled. (Courtesy of Drs. Janson, Martins, Henriques, de Freitas, Pinzan, and de Almeida of the University of São Paulo, Bauru Dental School, Brazil.)

Figure 288

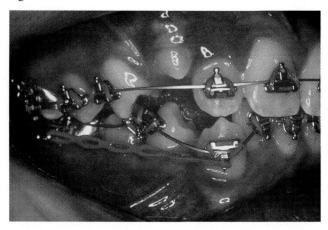

Figure 289

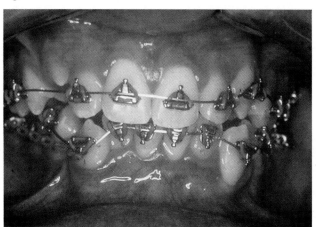

Figure 290

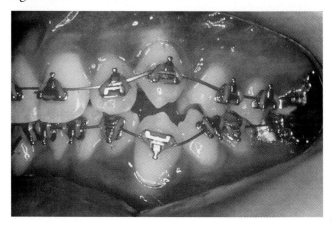

Figures 291–293

Three months later, note the significant improvement in leveling. The upper right canine has just erupted and was included in the system. (Courtesy of Drs. Janson, Martins, Henriques, de Freitas, Pinzan, and de Almeida of the University of São Paulo, Bauru Dental School, Brazil.)

Figure 291

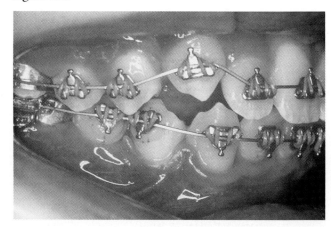

Section II: *Treatment*

Figure 292

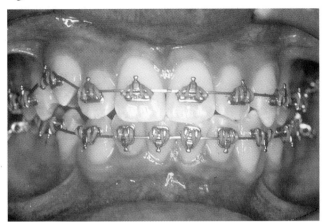

Figure 293

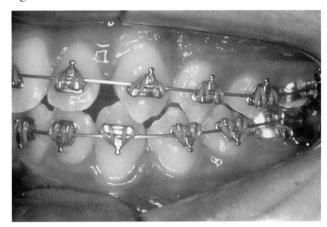

Figures 294–296

Toward the end of treatment, midline elastics improved inter-cuspation. (Courtesy of Drs. Janson, Martins, Henriques, de Freitas, Pinzan, and de Almeida of the University of São Paulo, Bauru Dental School, Brazil.)

Figure 294

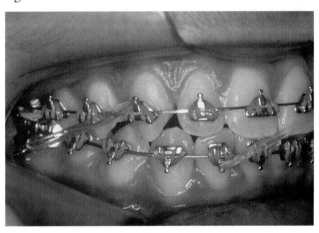

Figure 295

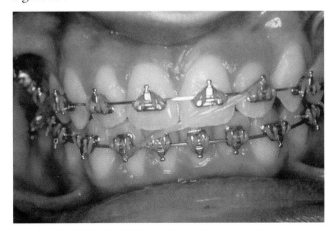

Figure 296

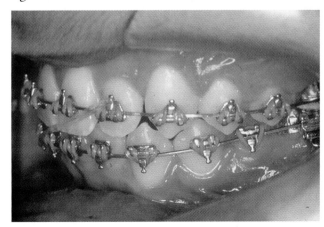

Figures 297–299

The patient finished after 14 months of treatment. Note the beautiful intercuspation and midline correction. (Courtesy of Drs. Janson, Martins, Henriques, de Freitas, Pinzan, and de Almeida of the University of São Paulo, Bauru Dental School, Brazil.)

Figure 297

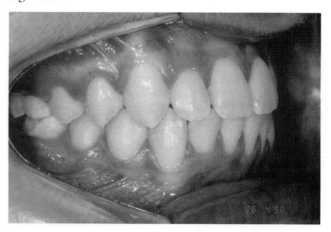

Figure 298

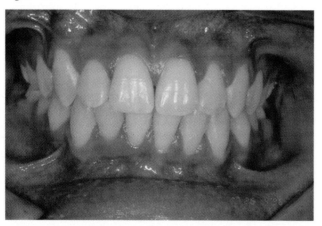

Figure 299

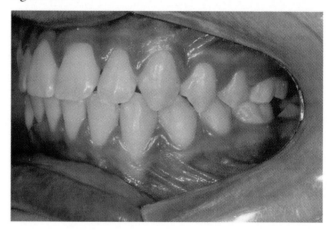

Figures 300–302

The patient in working and balancing canine guidance and anterior protrusion. The protection of the occlusion is excellent. (Courtesy of Drs. Janson, Martins, Henriques, de Freitas, Pinzan, and de Almeida of the University of São Paulo, Bauru Dental School, Brazil.)

Figure 300

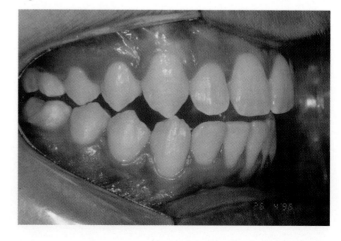

Section II: *Treatment*

Figure 301

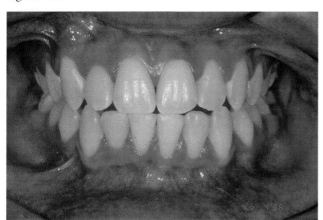

Figure 302

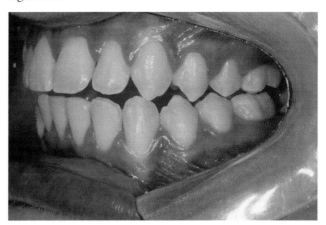

Figures 303, 304

Patient's facial and profile views after treatment. (Courtesy of Drs. Janson, Martins, Henriques, de Freitas, Pinzan, and de Almeida of the University of São Paulo, Bauru Dental School, Brazil.)

Figure 303

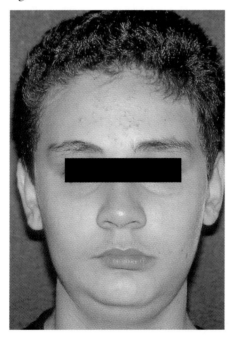

Figure 304

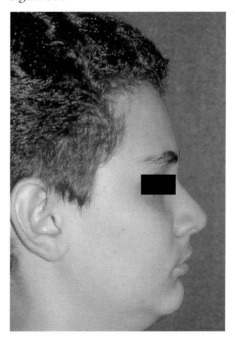

Figures 305, 306

Patient's cephalometric radiographs, before and after treatment. Note the improvement of the deep bite. (Courtesy of Drs. Janson, Martins, Henriques, de Freitas, Pinzan, and de Almeida of the University of São Paulo, Bauru Dental School, Brazil.)

Figure 305

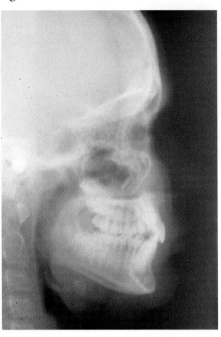

Figure 306

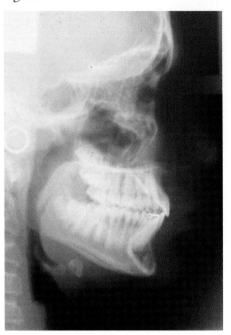

Figures 307, 308

Patient's panoramic radiographs before and after treatment. Note the beautiful root parallelism without root resorption. (Courtesy of Drs. Janson, Martins, Henriques, de Freitas, Pinzan, and de Almeida of the University of São Paulo, Bauru Dental School, Brazil.)

Figure 307

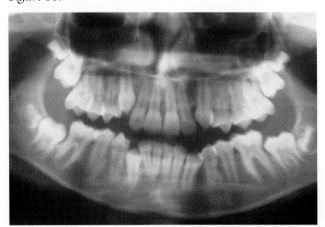

Figure 308

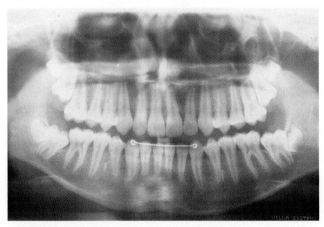

Figures 309, 310

This young man has a full upper lip and a convex profile. (Courtesy of Dr. Luiz Carlos de Mesquita Cabral.)

Figure 309

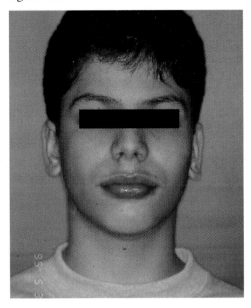

Figure 310

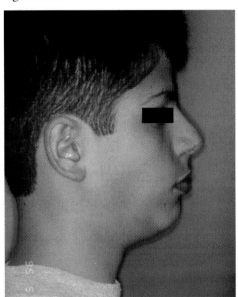

Figures 311, 312

The buccal and anterior views demonstrate a moderately deep bite. (Courtesy of Dr. Luiz Carlos de Mesquita Cabral.)

Figure 311

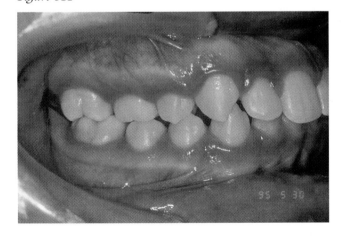

Figure 312

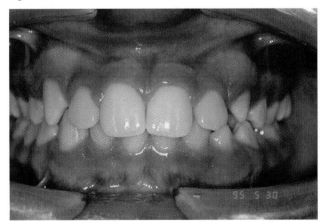

Figures 313, 314

The triangular brackets with a superelastic wire. (Courtesy of Dr. Luiz Carlos de Mesquita Cabral.)

Figure 313

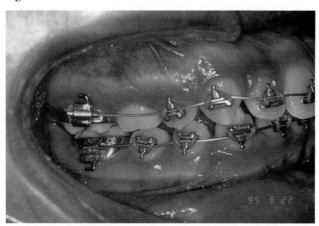

Figure 314

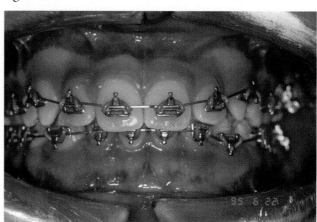

Figures 315, 316

Two months later, significant leveling has already taken place. (Courtesy of Dr. Luiz Carlos de Mesquita Cabral.)

Figure 315

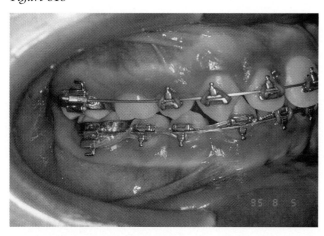

Figure 316

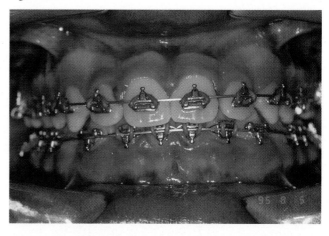

Figures 317, 318

The total treatment lasted about a year. Note the bite opening and the excellent leveling. The patient received only two sets of wires, a 16 × 22 superelastic, followed by a 16 × 22 stainless steel. (Courtesy of Dr. Luiz Carlos de Mesquita Cabral.)

Figure 317

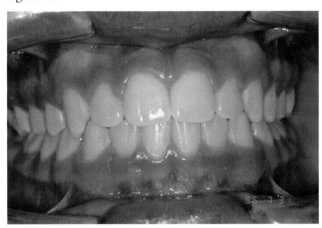

Figure 318

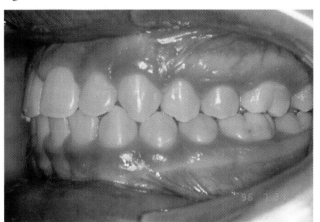

Figures 319, 320

Before and after cephalometric radiographs of the patient demonstrate excellent incisor inclinations and positions. (Courtesy of Dr. Luiz Carlos de Mesquita Cabral.)

Figure 319

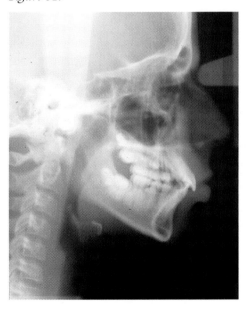

Figure 320

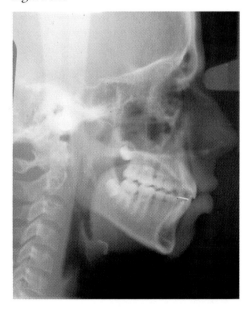

Figures 321, 322

Before and after panoramic radiographs demonstrate the excellent parallelism achieved with this contemporary therapy. Again, there are no signs of any resorption, thanks to the short treatment time. (Courtesy of Dr. Luiz Carlos de Mesquita Cabral.)

Figure 321

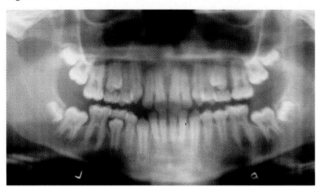

Figure 322

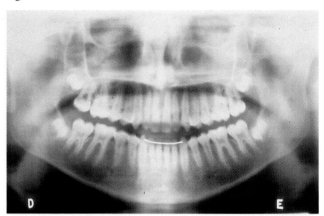

Figures 323–327

This young man is in his late mixed dentition, as demonstrated from the cephalometric and panoramic radiographs. He has a deep bite that can be alleviated nicely during the period of premolar eruption, so that by the time all the teeth are in the mouth, the case will be completed.

Figure 323

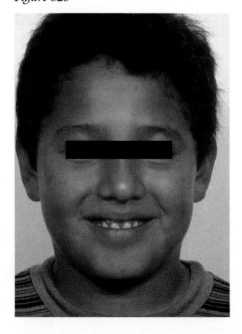

Figure 324

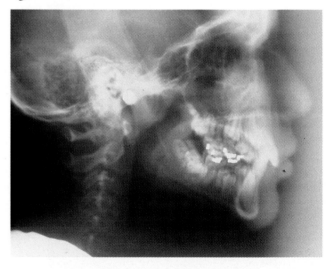

Figure 325

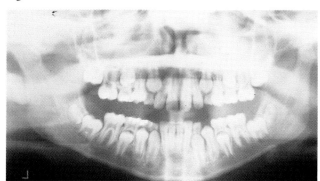

Figure 326

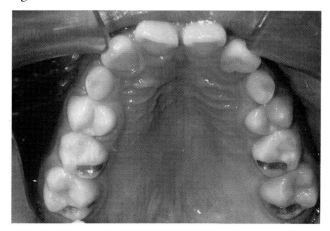

Figure 327

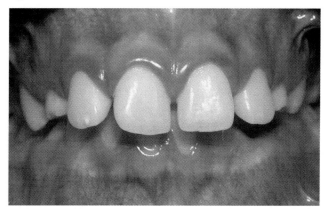

Figures 328, 329

Upper 2 × 2 and lower 2 × 4 intrusion arches were given. Note the double-tie configuration on the upper incisor. The wire has a tip back bend in front of the molar and is cinched back. The wire is 0.018-inch stainless steel.

Figure 328

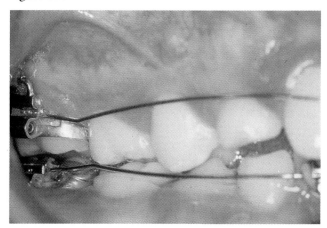

Figure 329

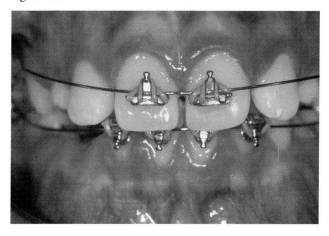

Figure 330

A few months later, after eruption of the premolars and canines, 20 × 20 superelastic wires are placed in the 0.022-inch slot brackets. The bite has opened significantly.

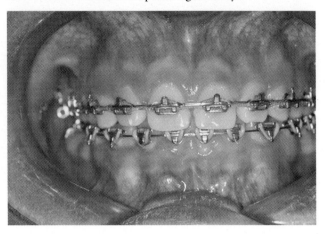

Figures 331–333

Toward the end of treatment, with the finishing 19 × 25 stainless steel wires in place. This sequence of mechanotherapy is another example of the efficiency of treatment that can be achieved while the natural permanent dentition is erupting into place, as mechanics and growth work in harmony together.

Figure 331

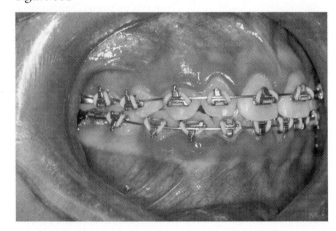

Figure 332

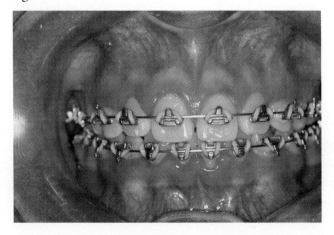

Figure 333

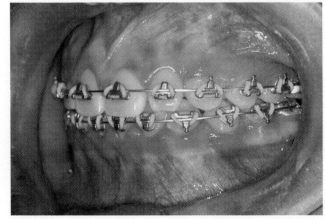

Section II: *Treatment*

Figures 334–338

This case is an example of the efficiency in leveling achieved with the new materials technology, as mild Class-II tendencies can easily be corrected with nonextraction into Class-I occlusions.

Figure 334

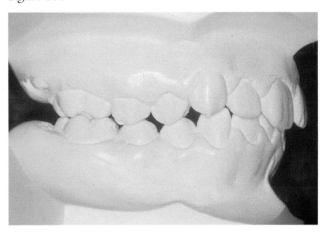

Figure 335

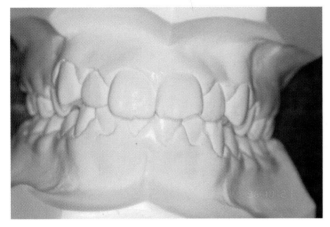

Figure 336

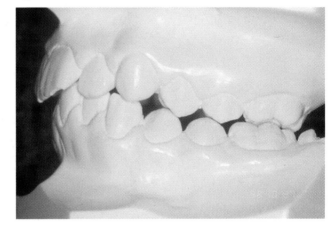

Figure 337

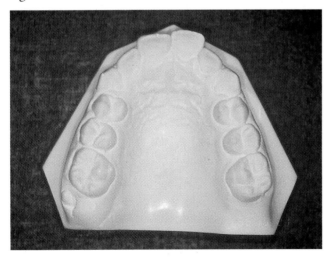

Figure 338

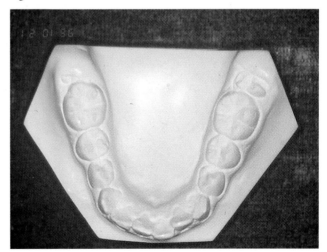

Figures 339–343

Same patient after just 1 year of treatment with the triangular brackets (0.022-inch slot) and only one set of 20 × 20 super-elastic wires. Note the perfect intercuspation, midline correction, and beautiful, broad dental arches.

Figure 339

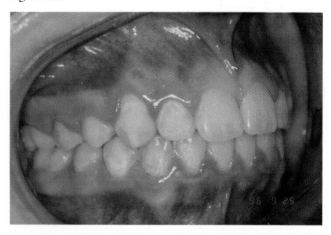

Figure 340

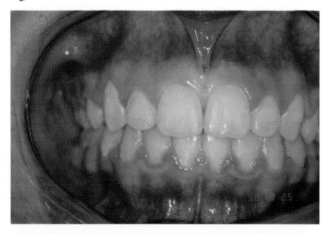

Figure 341

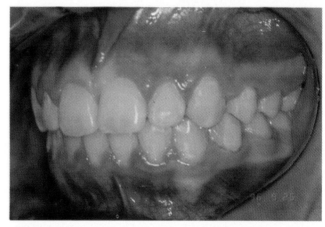

Figure 342

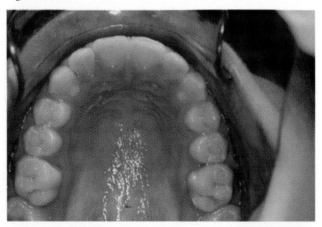

Figure 343

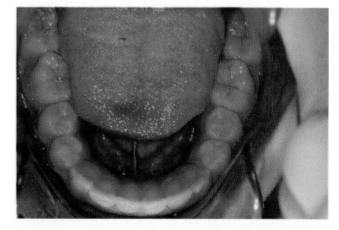

Figure 344

Patient's picture before treatment and just before the appliances were removed.

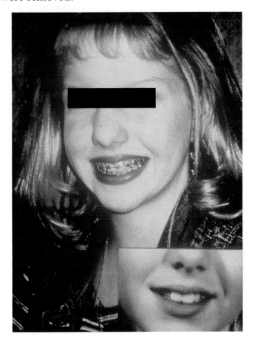

Figure 345

The patient now has a beautiful smile from corner to corner in just 1 year of fixed appliance therapy. The same case would have taken 2 or more years to complete, with numerous stainless steel wires.

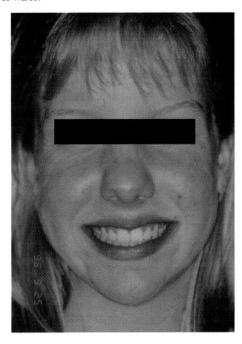

Figures 346–348

This patient had a Class-II, division 1 malocclusion with a 12-mm overjet.

Figure 346

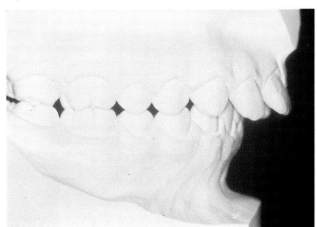

Figure 347

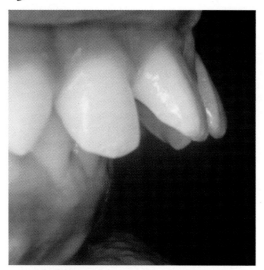

Figure 348

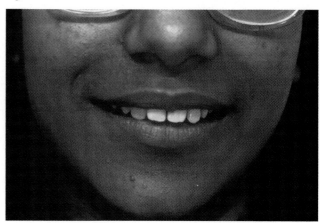

Figures 349–351

She was treated nonextraction by sequential distal movement of the posterior teeth into a Class-I relation using superelastic coil springs. The result is an excellent occlusion with a broad smile. It was achieved in approximately 2 years because distal movement of teeth is very time consuming.

Figure 349

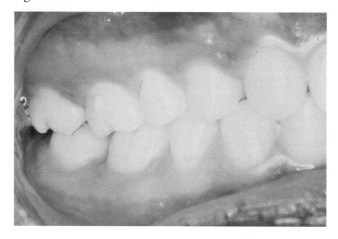

Figure 350

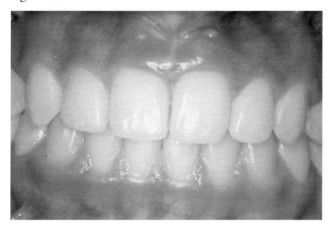

Figure 351

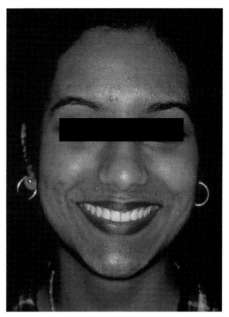

Figures 352, 353

The dramatic difference in the inclination of the teeth is shown clearly on the before and after cephalometric radiographs, demonstrating that the reduction in the overjet was accomplished through excellent control of teeth movement distally. Note the reduction of the upper lip procumbency as the upper incisors were brought into an upright position.

Figure 352

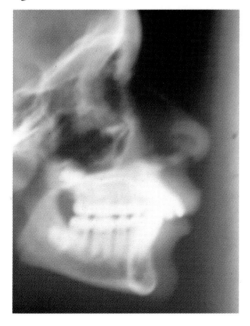

Figure 353

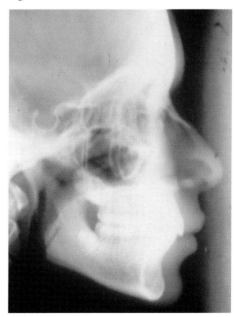

Figures 354, 355

The before and after panoramic radiographs demonstrate excellent root parallelism.

Figure 354

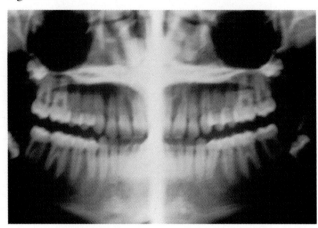

Figure 355

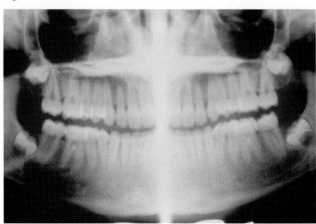

Figures 356–359

Three years later, the patient's occlusion has not changed even slightly. The patient wears her retainers only 12 hours a day, three times a week. Her smile is broad and the same as it was when treatment was completed.

Figure 356

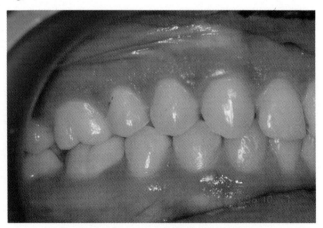

Figure 357

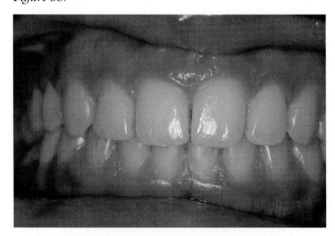

Figure 358

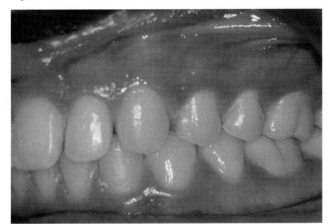

Figure 359

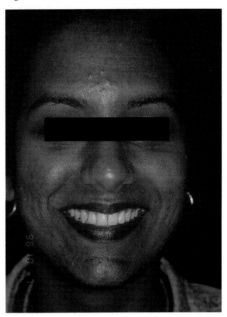

Figures 360, 361

The before and after appearance of a patient's profile when extractions of the upper first premolars were used and contemporary orthodontic mechanotherapy brought the upper incisors distally into the extraction site. Note the dramatic improvement of this patient's profile in just a year of treatment. This was accomplished in about half the time it took for the previous case. If the end results are going to be the same from an aesthetic and functional standpoint, then a shorter treatment time would be the therapy of choice. For most Class-II patients, the choice of treatment may well constitute a patient preference based on treatment time.

Figure 360

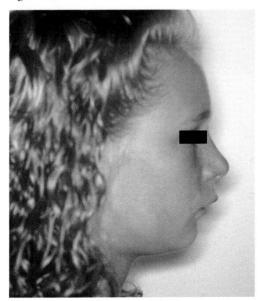

Figure 361

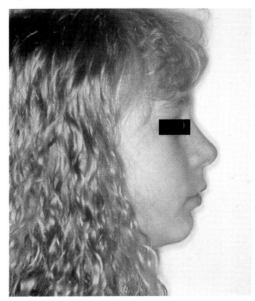

Tooth Recontouring Technique (TRT)

Mesial first molar—distal cuspid up to 3 mm/quadrant

Figures 362–364

Tooth recontouring is implemented in contemporary orthodontic mechanotherapy to bring the mesial and distal thicknesses of the posterior teeth enamel into their natural state, as if they had been worn down from a natural source of foods. Shown here is the lower jaw of a "patient" from ancient times, when flat proximal surfaces were common and crowded teeth uncommon (Figure 362). Note the natural contact surfaces. With today's eating habits, crowding has become a common factor in dentition (Figures 363, 364). By simulating the natural wear, we can obtain space to align the anterior teeth within the confines of the jaw.

Figure 362

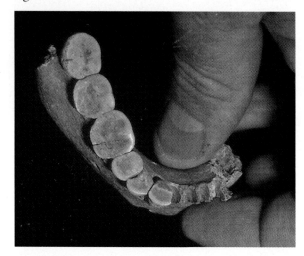

Figure 363

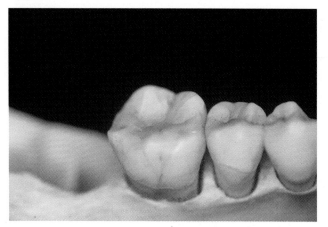

Figure 364

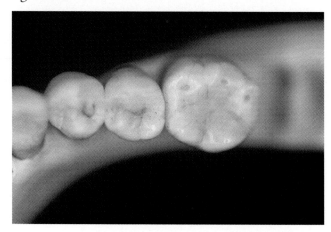

Section II: *Treatment*

Figures 365–368

This patient had inadequate space for the upper right lateral incisor. By recontouring the interproximal surfaces from molar to molar, enough space was obtained to align that tooth.

Figure 365

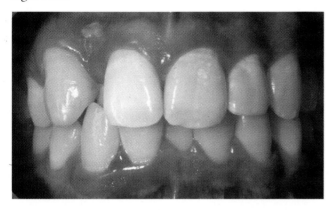

Figure 366

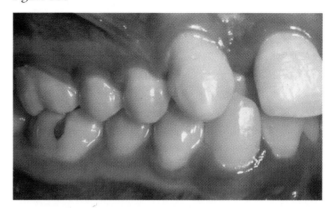

Figure 367

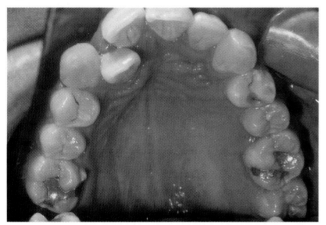

Figure 368

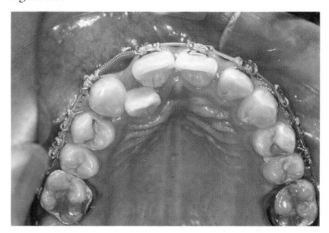

Figures 369, 370

Coil springs opened up space for the lateral incisor.

Figure 369

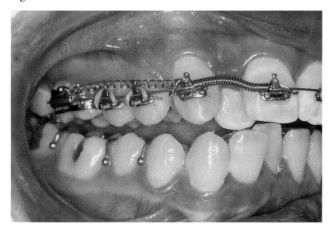

Figure 370

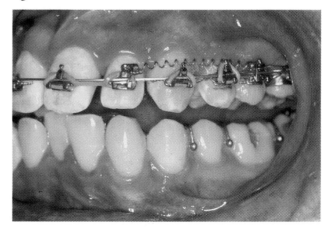

Figures 371, 372

The upper right lateral incisor is coming out of crossbite just a few months into treatment.

Figure 371

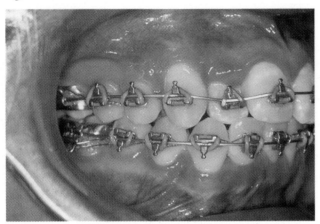

Figure 372

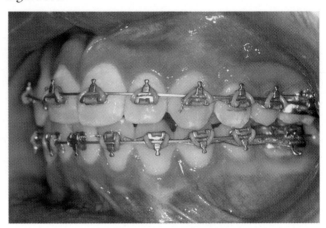

Figures 373, 374

The case was completed in approximately 1 year.

Figure 373

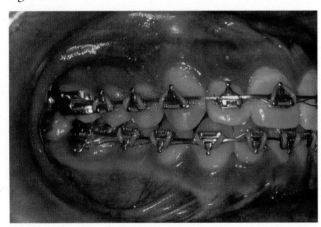

Figure 374

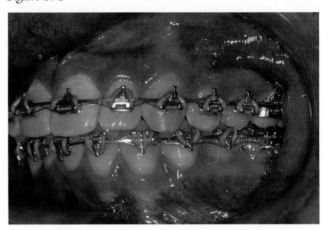

Figures 375–378

This woman demonstrated moderate upper and lower crowding with an open-bite tendency. She was treated with the old stainless steel mechanics. Today, she would have been treated with tooth recontouring. At the time, her clinician opted for extractions of the upper first premolars and the lower second premolars.

Figure 375

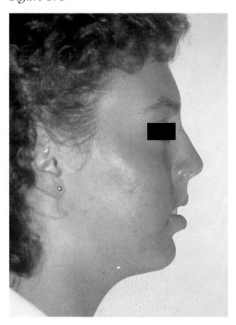

Figure 376

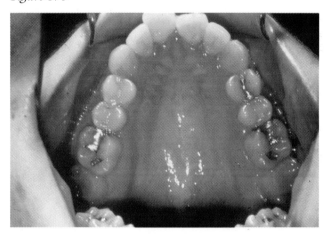

Figure 377

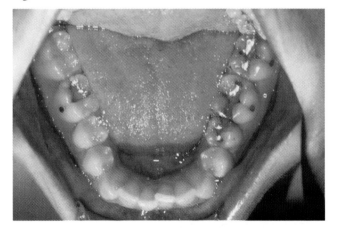

Figure 378

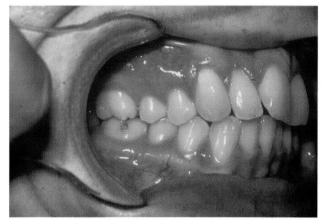

Figures 379–381

It took 6 months to obtain alignment and adequate leveling before space closure was initiated. Space closure was completed in about 18 months.

Figure 379

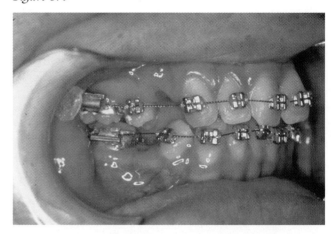

Figure 380

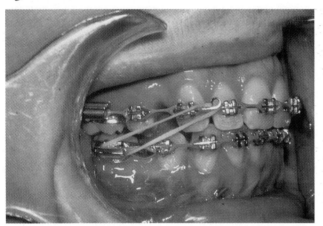

Figure 381

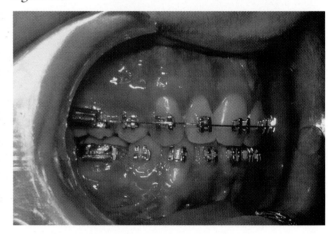

Figures 382–387

Appliances were removed after approximately 2 years of treatment. Note the upright position of the dentition, the narrow arches, and the somewhat flat profile of the patient. Not only did this case take unnecessarily long, but the extraction treatment was inappropriate because tooth recontouring would have resolved the crowding.

Figure 382

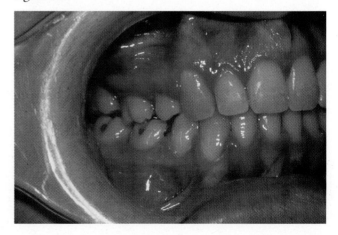

Figure 383

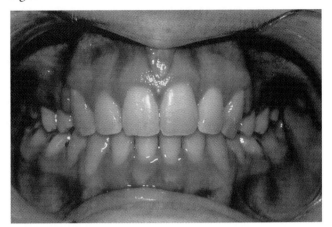

Figure 384

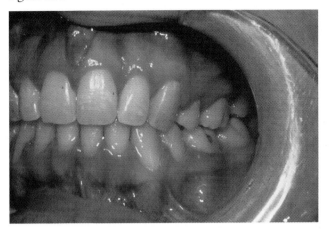

Figure 385

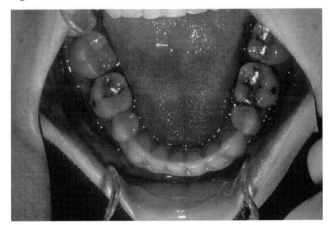

Figure 386

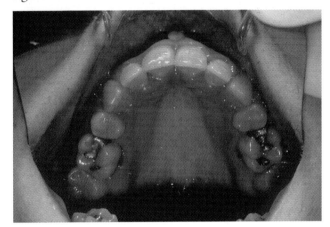

Figure 387

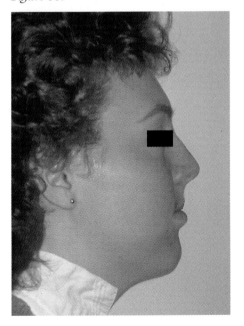

Figures 388–392

This young patient in the mixed dentition demonstrates a Class-II molar relation with narrow upper and lower arches, an open bite, procumbent upper incisors, and recession of the lower incisor soft tissue. Treatment plans in the mixed dentition for patients of this nature would involve broadening the arches with upper and lower expansion appliances.

Figure 388

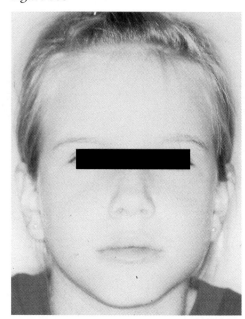

Figure 389

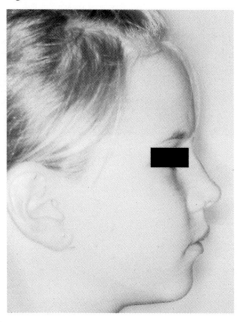

Figure 390

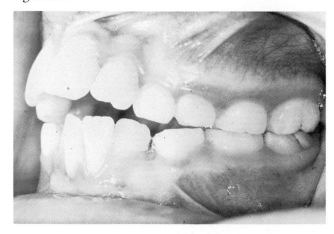

Figure 391

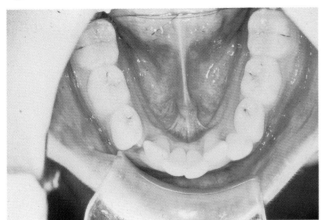

Figure 392

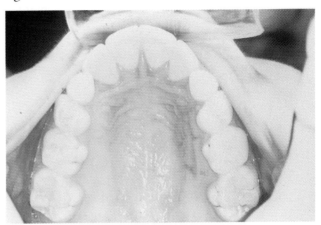

Figures 393–395

The upper expansion appliance is a Hyrax type, with bands on the molars and a wire configuration that extends to the primary canines. The screw is turned once a day for a month, at which point it is sealed and held for another month. The separation of the central incisor is due to the mid-palatal sutural opening. Two months later, the expander is removed and a 2 × 4 appliance (0.022-inch triangular brackets) with the 20 × 20 superelastic wire configuration aligns the incisors nicely.

Figure 393

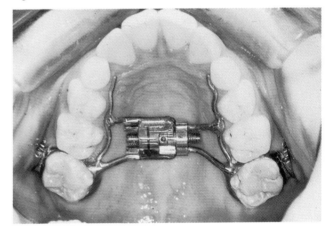

Figure 394

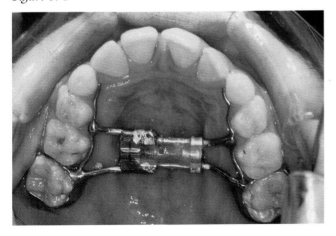

Figure 395

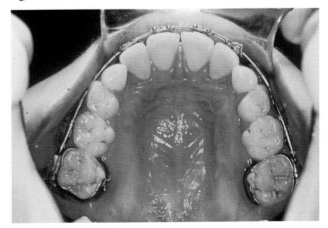

Expansion in the lower arch is attempted with a removable appliance. The screw is turned once a week for 6 to 7 months, until eruption of the lower permanent canines. As the canines erupt more buccally, the alveolar bone supports them, which may enhance the stability of the expansion. It is emphasized that expansion in the lower arch is dentoalveolar in nature, and not sutural. Therefore, it is imperative that it not be continued past the eruption of the lower canines because that may result in relapse of the inner canine width.

Figure 396

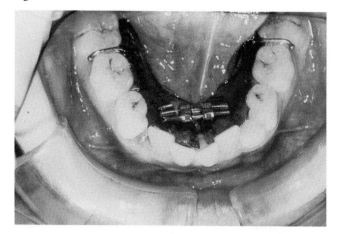

Figure 397

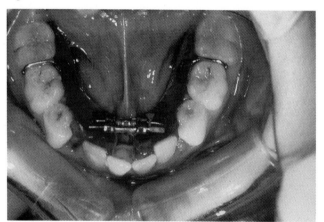

Figure 398

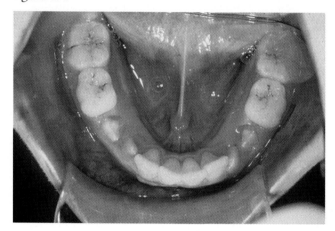

Figure 399

Just 8 months into treatment, the expansion has resulted in improvement of the Class-II relation into a Class-I molar relation, closure of the anterior open bite, and attainment of space for eruption of the remaining permanent teeth.

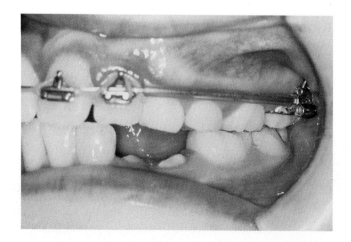

This series of photographs shows the patient before expansion, after a few months of expansion, and toward the end of treatment, as the permanent canines are erupting into position. Note the wonderful improvement in this patient's width of smile. Mixed dentition therapy in Class-II cases of this nature indeed results in dramatic improvement. Also note that the expansion did not result in further recession of the lower soft tissue. Periodontal grafting in that area was done before expansion. Had no mixed dentition expansion been attempted, extraction of permanent teeth would have been necessary with detrimental effects on this young girl's smile and happy demeanor.

Figure 400

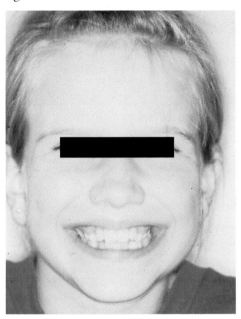

Figure 401

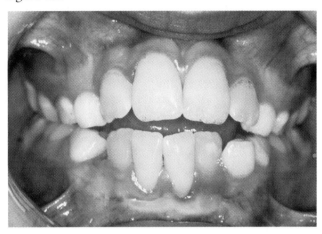

Figure 402

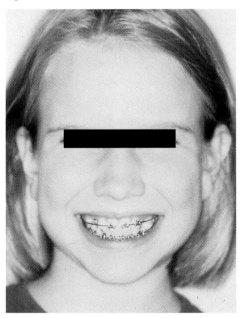

Figure 403

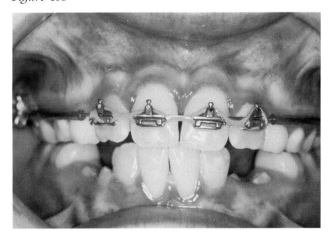

Figures 400–405 (continued)

Figure 404

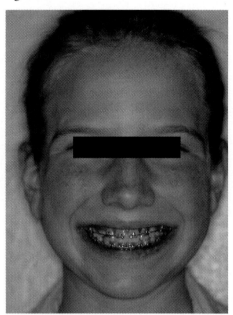

Figure 405

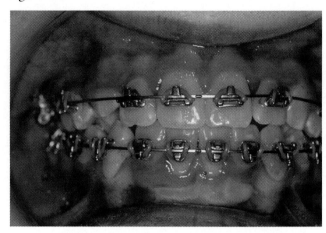

Figure 406

Maxillary deficiency occurs in a large percentage of Class-III skeletal malocclusions (20–50%). It is indicated by a straight vertical shadow from the infraorbital margin, through the alar base of the nose, to the corner of the mouth. The reverse-pull facemask in combination with a fixed palatal expansion appliance is proposed as the treatment method of choice for early interception of Class-III malocclusions. Treatment should begin as soon as the maxillary central and lateral incisors and maxillary first molars have completely erupted. Rapid palatal expansion can produce a slight forward movement of point A and a slight downward and forward movement of the maxilla. The effect of such expansion is to disrupt the maxillary sutural system, thus possibly enhancing the orthopedic effect of the facial mask by making sutural adjustments occur more readily. Several investigators have demonstrated the dramatic skeletal changes that can be obtained in animals with continuous protraction forces to the maxilla. The entire maxilla is displaced anteriorly, with significant effects as far posteriorly as the zygomaticotemporal suture. The facial mask is secured to the face by stretching elastics from the hooks on the maxillary splint to the crossbow of the facial mask. Heavy forces are generated, usually through the use of 5/8-inch, 14-oz elastics bilaterally. The current version of the facial mask is made of two pads that contact the soft tissue in the forehead and chin regions. Significant dentoskeletal changes and improvements in dentofacial profile result from 6 months of treatment with maxillary expansion and protraction. In instances in which no transverse change is necessary, the expansion appliance is activated once a day for a week to produce a disruption in the sutural system that facilitates the action of the facemask. A week later, the facemask therapy is initiated. The position of the crossbar is similarly adjusted in the vertical dimension to allow the elastics to pass through the interlabial gap without producing discomfort to the patient. The elastics travel in an inferomedial direction anteriorly from the hooks on the splint to the crossbar. If the tendency of an anterior open bite is suspected in a patient, an anterior site of protraction is required (premolar or even in front of the canine). Care must be taken that the elastics do not cause irritation to the corners of the mouth. The patient should wear the facemask on a full-time basis, except during meals. Young patients (5–9 years of age) can usually follow this regimen, particularly if the patient is told that full-time wear will last only 3 to 5 months. The patient should be seen every 8 to 12 weeks to check on the condition of the splint and to evaluate the hard and soft tissue changes. The facial mask is usually worn until a positive overjet of 2–4 mm is achieved interincisally. The possible treatment effects include a forward and

Figure 406 *(continued)*

downward movement of the maxilla, a forward and downward movement of the maxillary dentition, and a downward and backward redirection of mandibular growth. Although several investigators have claimed definite orthopedic advancement of the maxilla with reverse-pull mechanics, this is somewhat questionable because the same results have also been observed in patients who had only palatal expansion. The increase in maxillary length could also be attributed to growth.

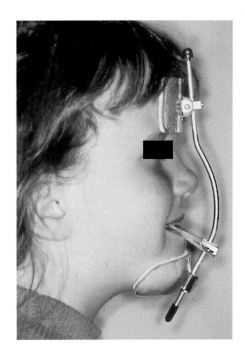

Figures 407–409

This boy with mixed dentition obtained a positive overbite and overjet relation after 6 months of reversed headgear therapy.

Figure 407

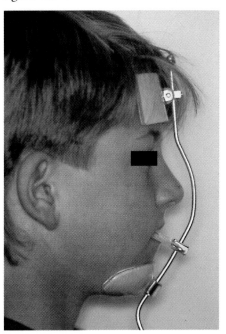

Figure 408

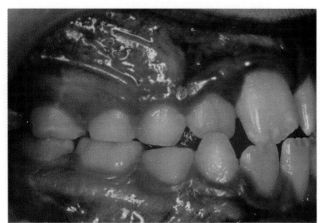

Figure 409

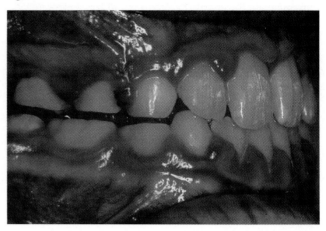

Figures 410, 411

True maxillary deficiency should not be confused with a pseudo-Class-III malocclusion, where the upper central incisors come in contact with the lower central incisors, and then the lower arch shifts forward into a negative overjet (underjet), giving the false appearance of a Class-III profile.

Figure 410

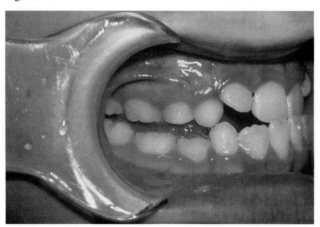

Figure 411

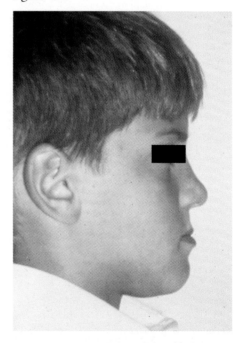

Figures 412, 413

The moment the upper incisors are tipped anteriorly with either fixed appliances or a spring retainer, the profile relation improves dramatically.

Figure 412

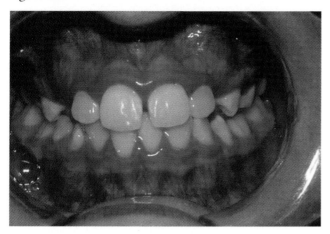

Figure 413

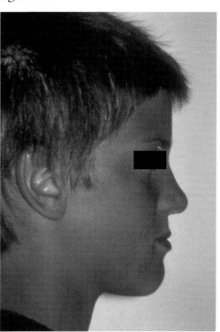

Figures 414–419

A maxillary deficiency should also not be confused with a true mandibular prognathism, where the lower arch is significantly broader than the upper and the posterior and the anterior teeth are tipped lingually. No contemporary treatment method can adequately control lower jaw growth. In other words, if the lower jaw "wants" to grow, it is going to grow no matter what. An orthognathic surgical procedure of mandibular setback after puberty would provide for a normal jaw and dental relation.

Figure 414

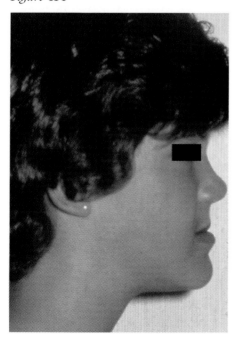

Figure 415

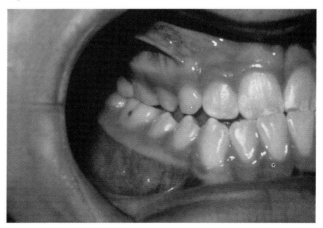

Figure 416

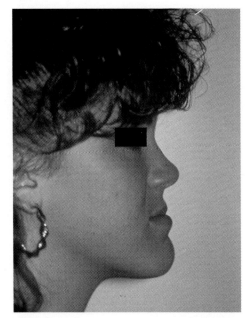

Figure 417

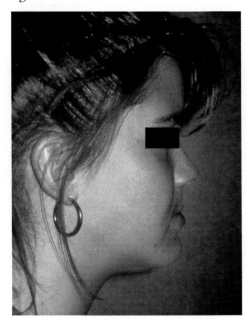

Figure 418

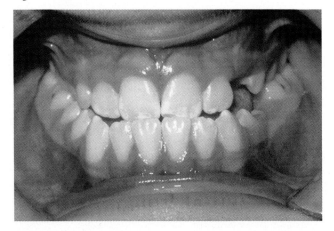

Figure 419

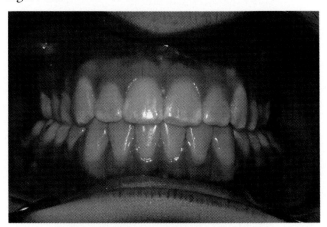

Extraction Therapy

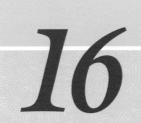

*I*t is simplistic and incorrect to blame undesirable facial esthetics after orthodontic treatment on the extraction of premolars. There is no predictable relation between the extraction of premolars and the esthetics of the smile. In reference to vertical changes after first premolar extractions, there are no significant differences between the vertical changes occurring in the extraction and nonextraction groups. On average, orthodontic treatment in both groups produced an increase in the cephalometric vertical dimensions that were examined. Retraction of the maxillary incisor was not significantly correlated with upper or lower lip vermilion height reduction. Retraction of the mandibular incisor was significantly correlated with lower lip vermilion height reduction (Figures 420–527).

The first objective of orthodontic mechanotherapy in the anteroposterior dimension is the attainment of a Class-I cuspid relation. This not only results in a stable, functional occlusion, but it ensures a good overbite and overjet relation when no tooth size discrepancy is present. The upper central and lateral incisor roots should be slightly convergent, and the remaining upper teeth should show a distal inclination, except for the second molars, which should be mesially tilted. The lower incisors should be upright, and the lower teeth should be increasingly distally inclined as one moves posteriorly.

In most instances, to obtain a Class-I cuspid relation, the cuspid tooth needs to move into the extraction space of the first bicuspid without loss of anchorage. All the clinician has to consider is the number of roots to be placed in opposition with each other in each unit. For example, if the posterior unit is composed of the first molar (three roots) and the second bicuspid (one root) and the anterior unit is composed of the cuspid (one large root) and the incisor teeth (two roots), we have a total of four posterior roots against three anterior roots. This will cause both units to move into the extraction space, thus resulting in anchorage loss. When, conversely, individual cuspid retraction is used (one anterior root) and the posterior unit is composed of the second and first molars and the second bicuspid (a total of seven posterior roots), it is easily seen that the cuspid tooth will move posteriorly almost without any anchorage loss (i.e., mesial movement of the upper posterior teeth).

Figures 420–425

This young woman has a bimaxillary protrusion of the dentition and a displeasing smile because of the blocked-out canines, and thus extraction of the first premolars would be the treatment of choice.

Figure 420

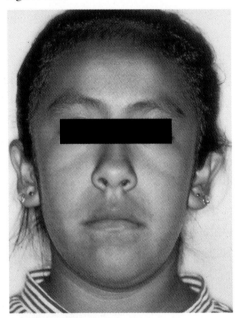

Figure 421

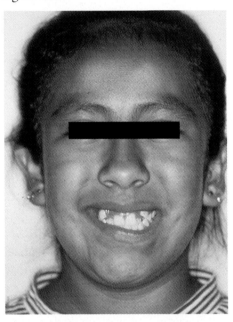

Figure 422

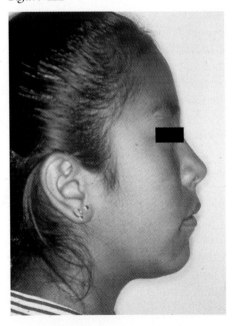

Figure 423

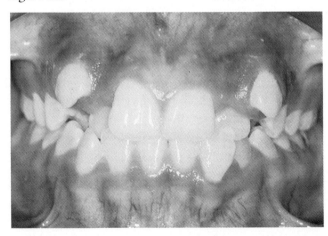

Figure 424

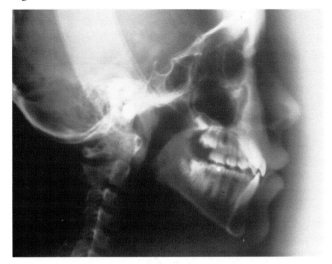

Figure 425

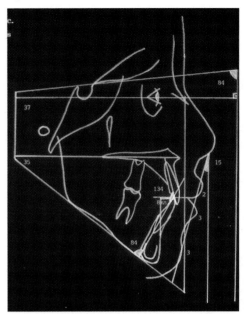

Figures 426–439

This series of slides shows the patient every 1 or 2 months. Her treatment was completed in a little over a year, and most of the time was spent in finishing and detailing the occlusion. The space closure was accomplished within a few months. The upper first premolar was extracted first and the upper canine was retracted into the extraction site within just 1 month of treatment with retraction of the upper coil spring. The lower first premolar was used as a reference. Two months into treatment, the lower premolar was also extracted, and the lower canine was retracted distally within the first 8 months of treatment. Note the bodily movement of the lower canine along the superelastic wire as the distal elbow of the bracket contacts the wire. The movement is similar to that of a children's see-saw. As soon as the crown tips a little, the distal elbow of the bracket will contact the wire, at which point crown movement will cease. The single slot, X_1, has become a wide twin slot, X_2. As soon as that is created, the root is uprighted. As soon as the root uprights, the X_2 slot becomes X_1. Immediately afterward, the crown will move and the distal elbow will contact the wire again, and the X_1 slot will again become X_2, and so forth. Note the panoramic radiograph: There is beautiful root parallelism from the beginning of treatment and root movement of the lower canines. As soon as a Class-I canine relation is established, elastomeric chains on a stainless steel wire finish the space closure. Finishing elastics aid in improvement of the intercuspation. After careful checking of the occlusal contacts, balancing and working canine guidance, and protrusive movements, the fixed appliances are removed. The movement was initiated on a 20×20 superelastic wire in the 0.022-inch bracket slot and finished with 19×25 stainless steel wires during the final stages of space closure. If the 0.018-inch slot had been used, this could have been accomplished using 16×22 wires.

Figure 426

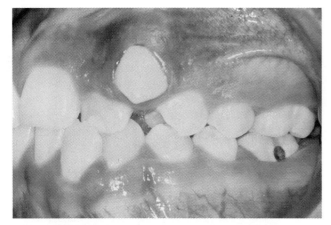

Figure 427

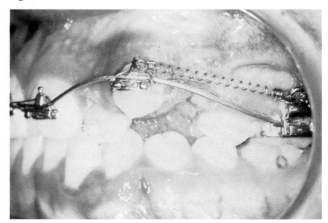

Figure 428

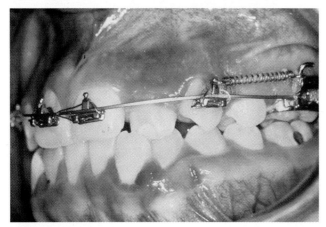

Figure 429

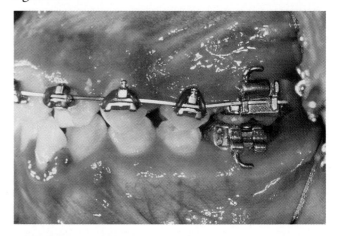

Figure 430

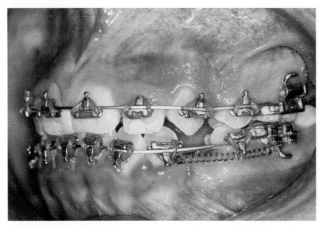

Figure 431

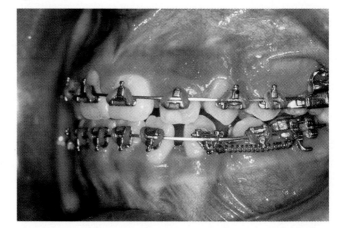

Figure 432

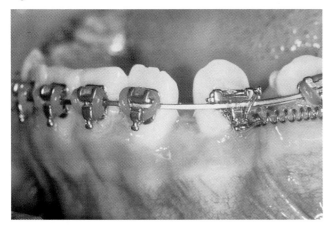

Figure 433

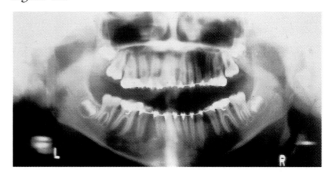

Figure 434

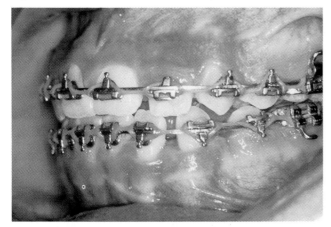

Figure 435

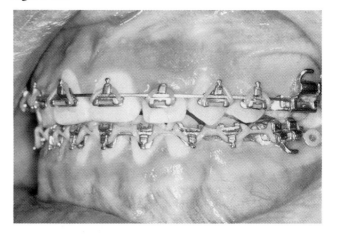

Figure 436

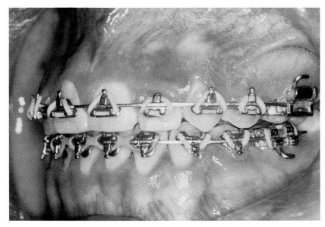

Figure 437

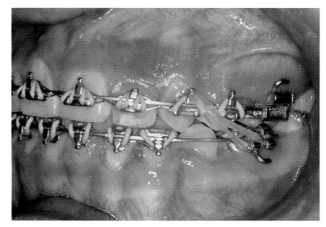

Figure 438

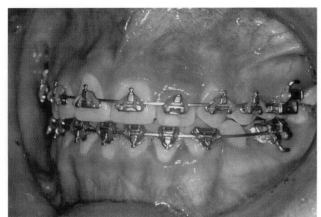

Figure 439

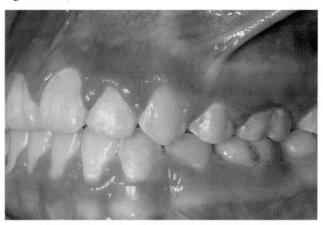

Figures 440–445

The same patient after treatment. Notice the nice, rounded arches that complement her smile line, and notice the midline correction and good intercuspation. Also note the improvement of her soft tissue profile. Periodontal plastic recontouring (see Section III, Chapter 19, on cosmetic dentistry) was recommended to the patient as part of her cosmetic dental enhancement.

Figure 440

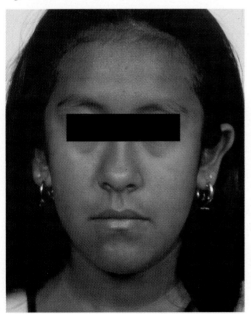

Figure 441

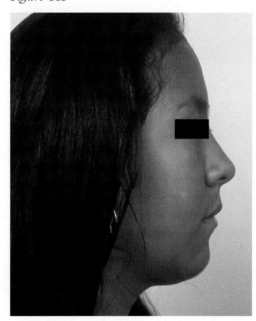

Figure 442

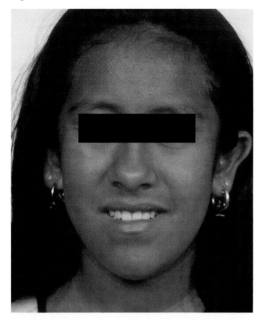

Figure 443

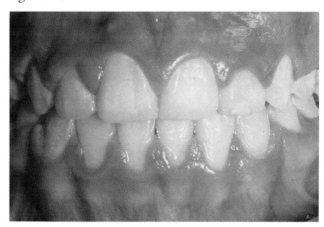

Figure 444

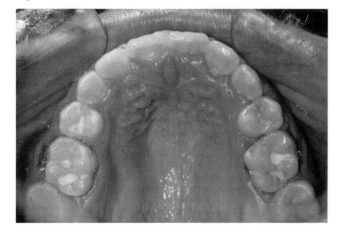

Figure 445

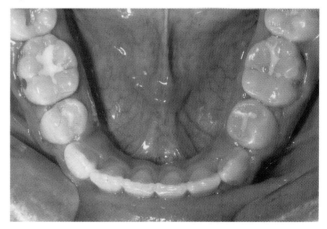

This adult patient had moderate upper and lower crowding and full soft tissue thickness.

Figure 446

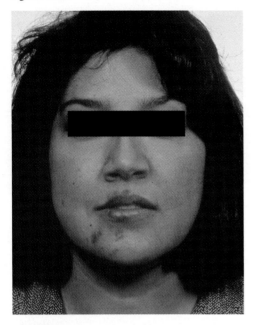

Figure 447

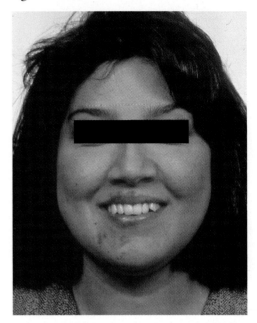

Figure 448

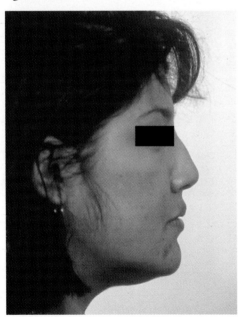

Figure 449

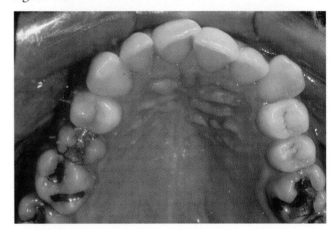

Figure 450

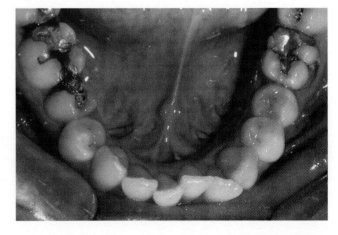

Figures 451–453

She had Class-I relation, moderate crowding and a slight open-bite tendency. Extractions of the upper and lower second premolars was the treatment of choice, followed by fixed appliances and retention.

Figure 451

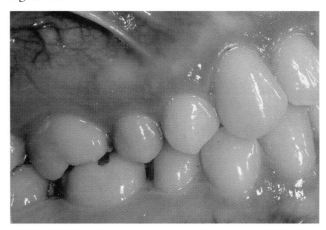

Figure 452

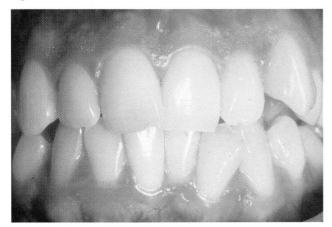

Figure 453

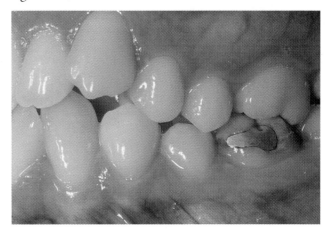

Figures 454–456

Triangular brackets with a superelastic wire (20 × 20 in the 0.022-inch slot or 16 × 22 in the 0.018-inch slot) can be used as initial archwires. Elastomeric chains can aid in the retraction of the first premolars into the extraction site.

Figure 454

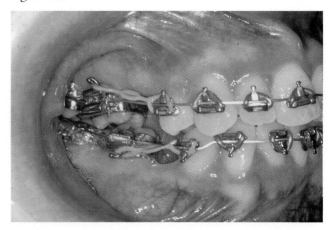

Figure 455

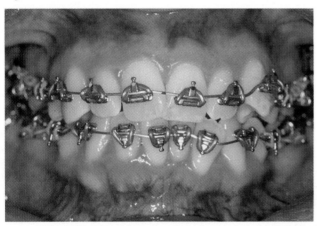

Figure 456

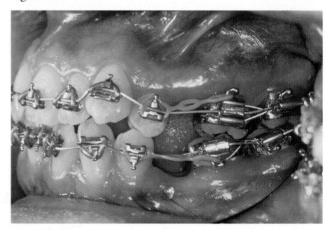

Figures 457–459

Superelastic coil springs were given at the following appointment to continue space closure.

Figure 457

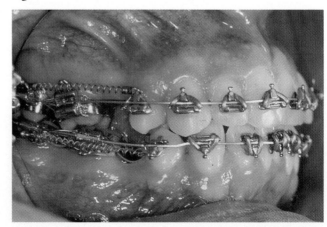

Figure 458

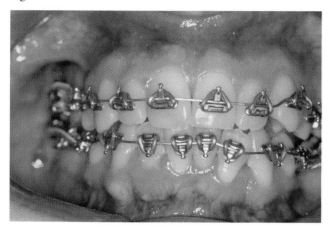

Figure 459

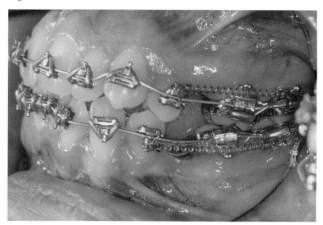

Figures 460–462

Within the first 6 months of treatment, significant alignment leveling and space closure has been accomplished.

Figure 460

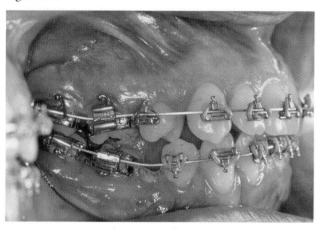

Figure 461

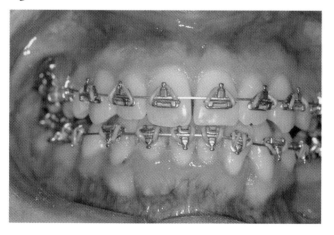

Figure 462

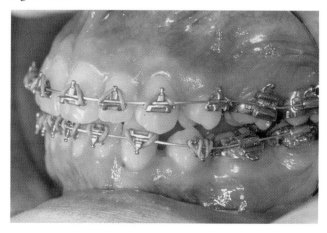

Figures 463–465

Because the canine and incisor teeth are now in better alignment, overall space closure is initiated. This can be done on the superelastic wire or on the stainless steel wire (19 × 25 in the 0.022-inch slot or 16 × 22 in the 0.018-inch slot)

Figure 463

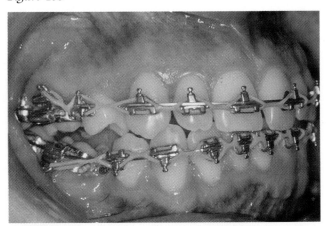

Figure 464

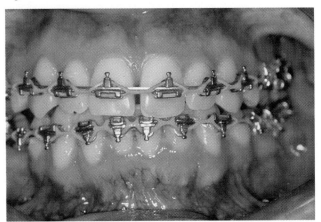

Figure 465

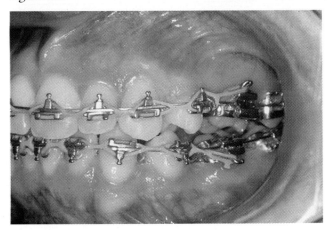

Figures 466–469

In about a year, as the patient approaches the end of therapy, a beautiful occlusion has developed with excellent intercuspation, midline correction, and a beautiful smile from corner to corner.

Figure 466

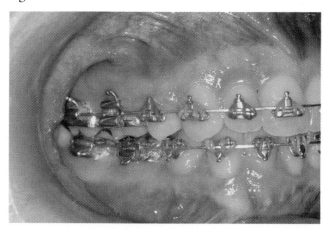

Figure 467

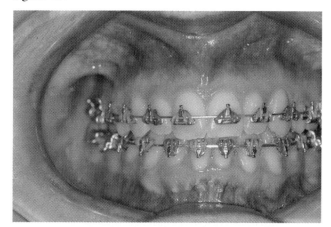

Figure 468

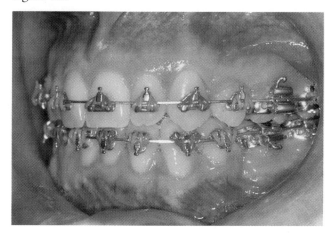

Figure 469

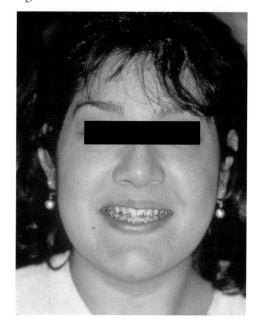

This young woman had a significant malocclusion of severe crowding. Because of the decayed lower first molars, an extraction therapy of the upper first canines and the lower first molars was chosen as the therapy. *premolars*

Figure 470

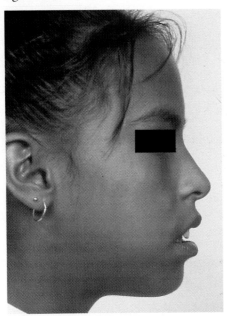

Figure 471

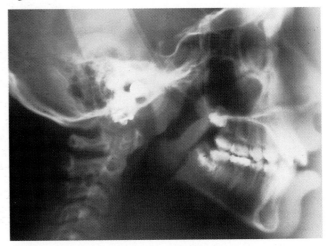

Figure 472

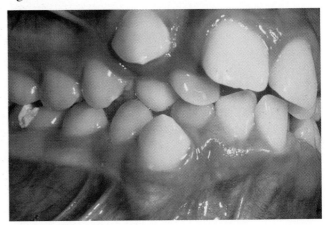

Figures 473–477

In the upper arch, the upper first premolars were removed. Within 2 months of treatment, the upper canines were retracted distally, and within 4 months of treatment the lateral incisors were being brought labially. Within the first 8 months of treatment the upper arch was beautifully aligned. The fast and easy movement shown here was once again accomplished because of the lower friction provided by the triangular brackets and the superelastic behavior of the new wire and coil springs. A single wire was used throughout this arch alignment.

Figure 473

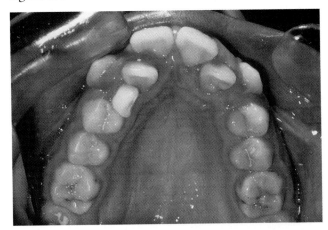

Figure 474

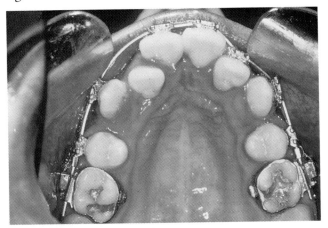

Figure 475

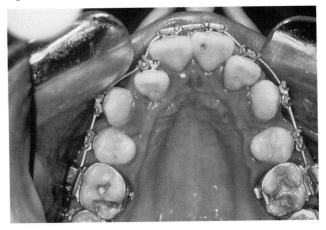

Figure 476

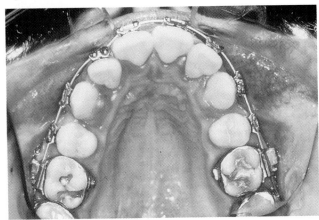

Figure 477

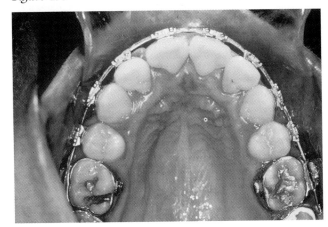

In the lower arch the first molars were extracted because of the poor long-term prognosis of those teeth. Space closure in the lower arch was accomplished within just 7 months, as shown clearly on the panoramic radiographs. Note that this is one of the toughest areas of the jaws for tooth movement over a long span of bone. Notice the excellent root parallelism and healthy bone formation and the absence of any signs of root resorption because the triangular brackets provide for an almost friction-free environment for easy sliding mechanics. The space closure was initially attempted on segmental wires, but these caused the second molars to tip a bit and were quickly abandoned. A continuous superelastic wire, followed by stainless steel, completed the movement. It is noteworthy that the bone physiology as well as the roots on the panoramic radiograph 7 months into this space closure appear to be in perfect health. Fast movement under light, continuous, biologic forces in a friction-free environment greatly enhances the efficient movement of teeth.

Figure 478

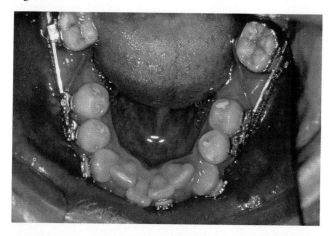

Figure 479

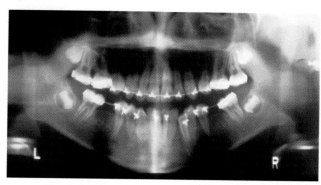

Figure 480

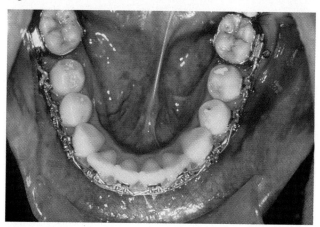

Figure 481

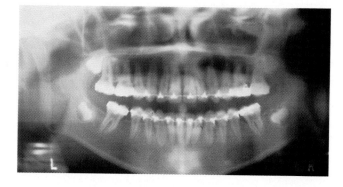

This patient's therapy was completed within 17 months of treatment. Note the beautiful intercuspation of teeth and the root parallelism on the final panoramic radiograph.

Figure 482

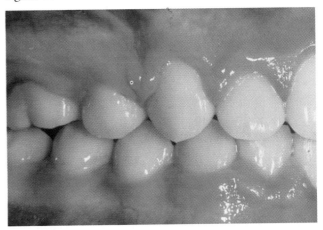

Figure 483

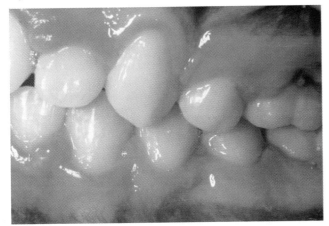

Figure 484

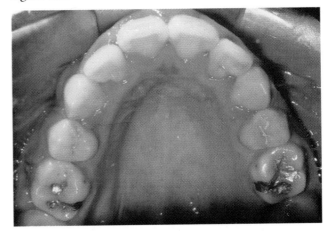

Figure 485

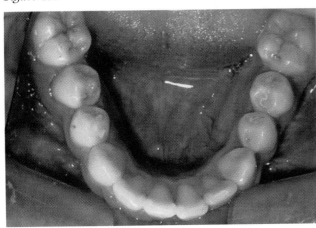

Figure 486

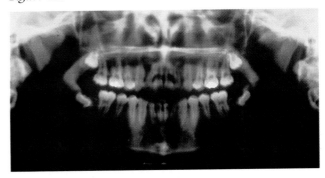

This adult patient had a Class-II retrognathic mandible and a Class-II dental malocclusion, upright incisors, deep overbite, and blocked-out upper canines. She refused any kind of surgery, and therefore an upper first premolar extraction therapy was the treatment of choice. (Courtesy of Dr. Luiz Carlos de Mesquita Cabral.)

Figure 487

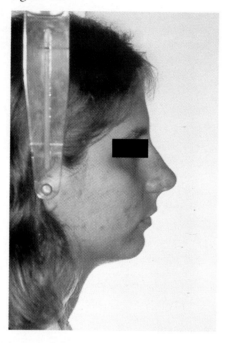

Figure 488

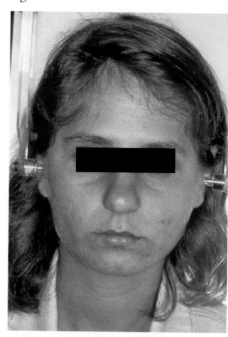

Figure 489

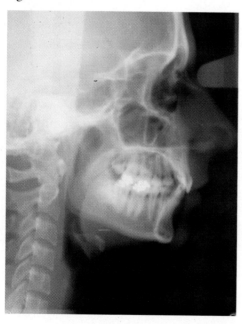

Figure 490

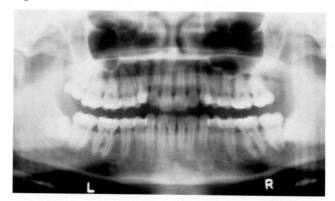

Figure 491

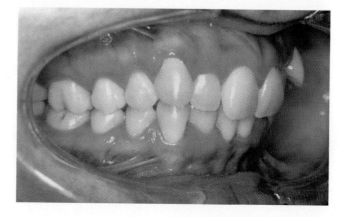

Figures 487–493 (continued)

Figure 492

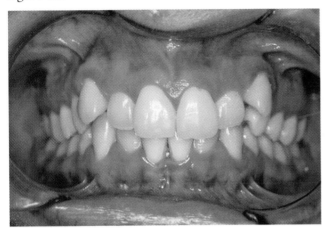

Figure 493

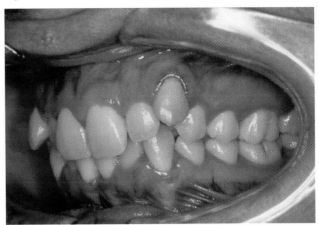

Figures 494–496

A superelastic wire was used in the triangular bracket slot with superelastic coil springs to retract the upper canines into a Class-I relation. (Courtesy of Dr. Luiz Carlos de Mesquita Cabral.)

Figure 494

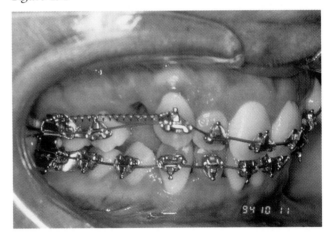

Figure 495

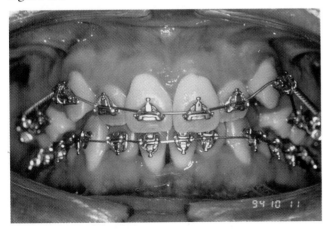

Figure 496

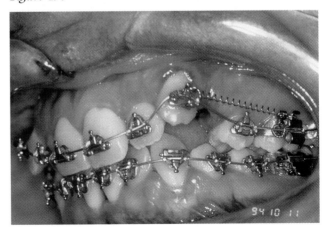

Two months into treatment, the canines have been retracted considerably. (Courtesy of Dr. Luiz Carlos de Mesquita Cabral.)

Figure 497

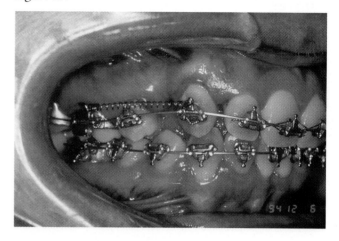

Figure 498

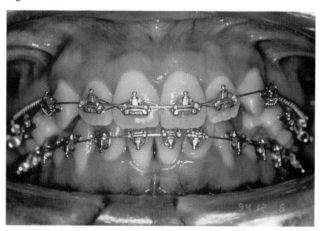

Figure 499

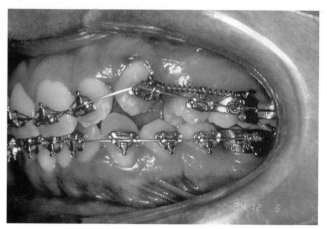

Figures 500–502

Three months into treatment, a Class-I canine relation has been achieved. (Courtesy of Dr. Luiz Carlos de Mesquita Cabral.)

Figure 500

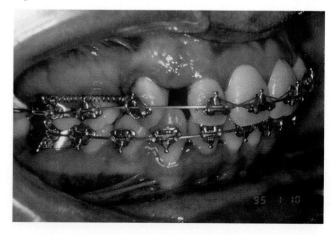

Figure 501

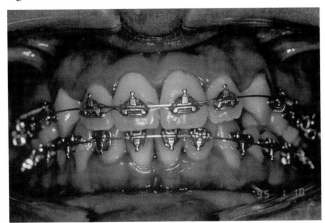

Figure 502

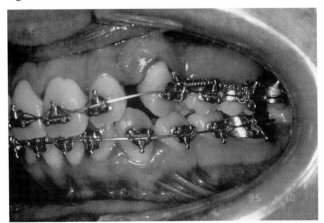

Figures 503–505

Four months into treatment, the torque of the upper incisors has been improved considerably. (Courtesy of Dr. Luiz Carlos de Mesquita Cabral.)

Figure 503

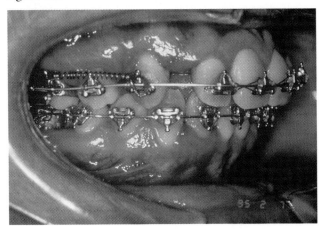

Figure 504

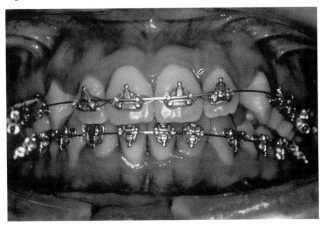

Figure 505

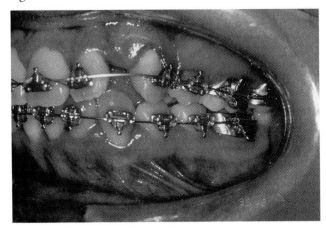

Figures 506–508

Ten months into treatment, superelastic coil springs are used to retract the upper incisors. (Courtesy of Dr. Luiz Carlos de Mesquita Cabral.)

Figure 506

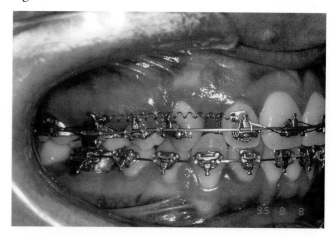

Figure 507

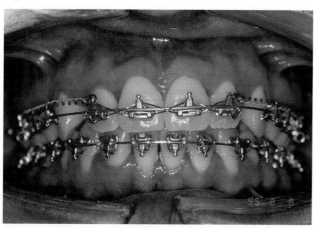

Figure 508

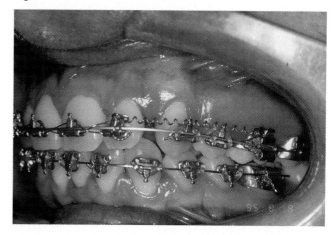

Figures 509–511

A year into treatment, the upper incisor torque is still being improved as the patient enters the final stages of treatment. (Courtesy of Dr. Luiz Carlos de Mesquita Cabral.)

Figure 509

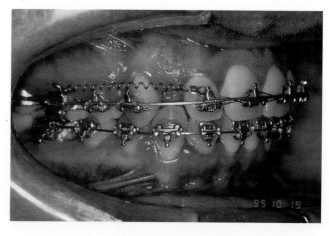

Figure 510

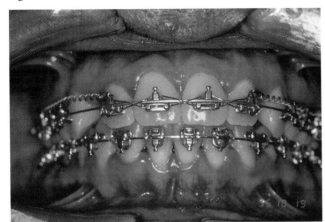

Figure 511

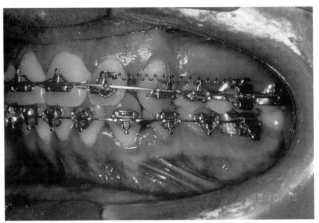

Figures 512–517

The fixed appliances were removed after 21 months of treatment. The patient's personal circumstances resulted in a delay in her treatment during the course of therapy. Note the improvement of the incisor root positions on the cephalometric radiograph, the beautiful root parallelism on the panoramic radiograph, and the improvement in the patient's facial and profile appearance. The space between the upper right canine and lateral incisor is a result of a tooth size discrepancy. Cosmetic dental bonding will be done to address the discrepancy in that area. (Courtesy of Dr. Luiz Carlos de Mesquita Cabral.)

Figure 512

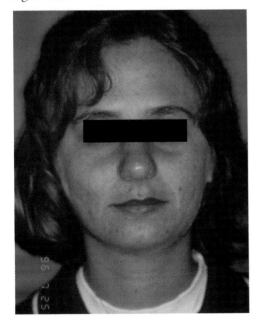

Figure 513

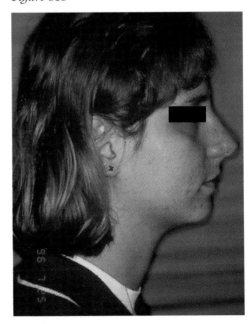

Figure 514

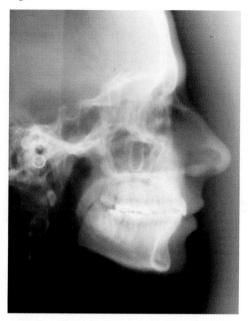

Figure 515

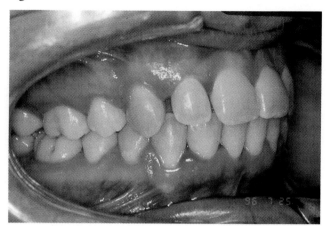

Figure 516

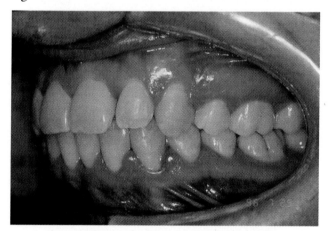

Figure 517

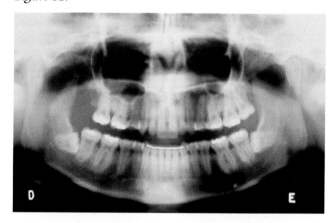

Figures 518–520

This young patient has a Class-II malocclusion, a deep bite, malformed upper second premolars, and crowding of the arches. As shown in the previous case, such malocclusions can be treated successfully with upper premolar extractions.

Figure 518

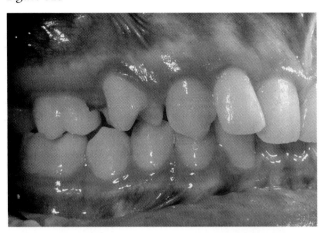

Figure 519

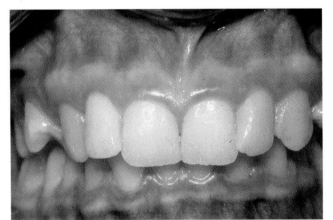

Figure 520

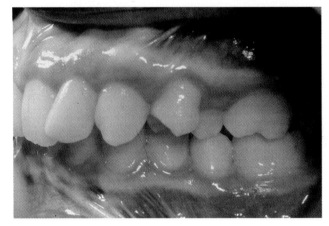

Figures 521, 522

Extraction of the malformed upper second premolars alleviated the crowding in the upper arch. Superelastic wires and triangular brackets provide the control needed to align levels and close spaces simultaneously.

Figure 521

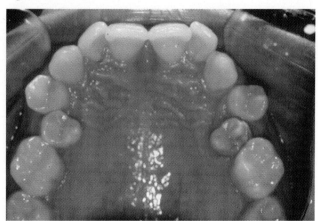

Figure 522

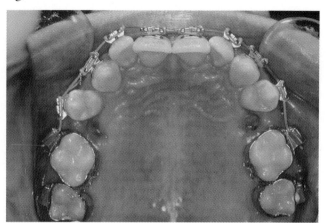

Figures 523, 524

To open the bite rapidly, a biteplate, with a groove in it to allow for a comfortable habitual position of the lower incisors and the biteplate apparatus, is used in the upper arch. The biteplate holds the sagittal position and allows the lateral open bites to improve naturally. The opening of the bite in the premolar region allows for the rapid extrusion of the premolars in that area with a 20 × 20 superelastic wire in the 0.022-inch bracket slot.

Figure 523

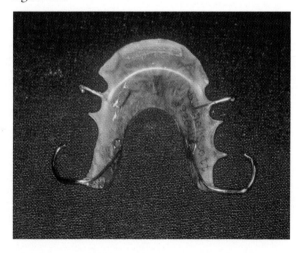

Figure 524

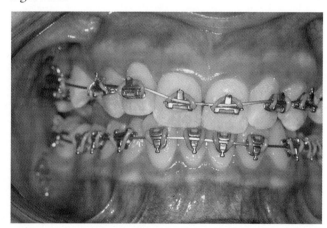

Figure 525

Two months into treatment, the biteplate is no longer necessary because the bite has opened adequately.

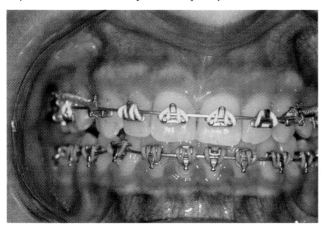

Figures 526, 527

Over the next few months of treatment, and in less than a year, with the alignment leveling, the bite opening, and the space closure completed, the patient is close to finishing treatment.

Figure 526

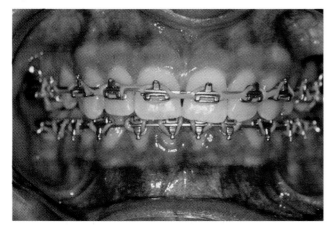

Figure 527

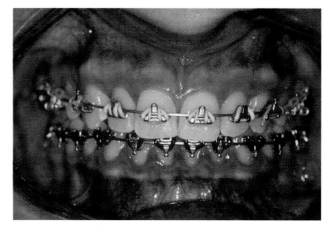

Posttreatment Considerations

III

Functional Occlusion and Occlusal Adjustment

Guilherme RP Janson, Décio Rodrigues Martins,
José Fernando Castanha Henriques, Marcos Roberto de Freitas,
Amaldo Pinzan, and Renato Rodrigues de Almeida

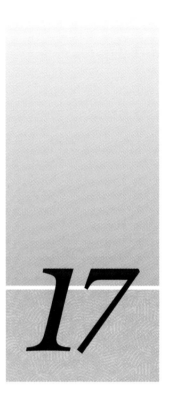

The Importance of the Centric Relation in Orthodontics

In orthodontics, diagnosis and treatment planning should be performed by an evaluation of the malocclusion with the mandible in centric relation (CR), that is, the natural musculoskeletal position of the condyle in the fossa, in order to obtain the true maxillary–mandibular skeletal and dental relations in the three planes of space. If this is overlooked, an incorrect diagnosis and treatment plan of the actual malocclusion, along with its unfavorable consequences, may result. Examples of this incorrect diagnosis include the case of a false Class-III that may incorrectly be considered a true Class-III, with a consequently poorer prognosis, or the case of a unilateral posterior crossbite that is, in fact, a bilateral cusp-to-cusp crossbite, in CR. Therefore, bilateral manipulation of the mandible into CR is imperative at the first visit. Any discrepancy should be recorded for later use during diagnosis and treatment planning. As usual, the models are trimmed and the lateral cephalometric headplates are obtained in centric occlusion because of the difficulties in taking them in CR. Hence, during treatment planning, the orthodontist has to consider any discrepancy presented. Moreover, during every appointment the patient has to be monitored in CR so that the mechanotherapy is guided to accomplish the final ideal static and functional occlusion with the mandible in this position. If this is disregarded, treatment may finish with the mandible in centric occlusion, with several prematurities that may later cause traumatic occlusion or craniomandibular disorders (Figures 528–552).

Problems Associated with Prematurities and Interferences

A premature contact or an interference characterizes a functional malocclusion. When the associated influence of a functional malocclusion with a certain level of emotional stress is higher than the individual physiologic tolerance, muscle hyperactivity is increased. When the forces produced by the muscle hyperactivity are higher than the structural tolerance, the structure with the smaller tolerance level will collapse. A prematurity or an interference, associated with stress, may cause a disorder in one of the following structures: teeth, periodontal structures, masticatory musculature, or TMJs. The weakest structure will collapse. For this reason, any prematurity must be eliminated at the end of orthodontic treatment. If the teeth present the smaller tolerance level, they may manifest occlusal wear or pericementitis. If the peridontium is the weakest structure, the teeth will present with mobility, alveolar bone loss, and gingival recession. If the musculature is the predominant structure involved, it will present with pain or dysfunction. When the TMJ is the primary structure involved, it may present with a wide range of disorders, depending on the severity of the prematurity as well as the length of time it has been present. Prematurities do not correct spontaneously because teeth are only momentarily in contact during function, and after some time they are the structures that may become compromised. It is unrealistic to expect a self-correction of prematurities and interferences after orthodontic therapy, because they may lead to craniomandibular dysfunction with all the consequent symptoms.

Orthodontic Treatment Objectives

The orthodontic treatment objectives are to provide good facial esthetics, and an ideal static and functional occlusion. The static objectives are Andrews' Six Keys to Normal Occlusion. The functional objectives are obtained with the mutually protected occlusion, which presents the following characteristics: (1) the teeth should present maximum intercuspation with the mandible in CR; (2) in CR, all posterior teeth should present effective occlusal contacts through their long axes and the anterior teeth should present a 0.005-inch clearance; (3) during lateral functional movements of the mandible, the cuspid should disclude all posterior teeth (cuspid guidance); (4) during protrusion, the six upper anterior teeth should articulate with the six lower anterior teeth and first or second premolars (in first premolar extraction cases) in order to disclude all the posterior teeth; and (5) there should be no balancing side interferences. This relation of the anterior teeth is known as anterior guidance.

Establishing a cuspid guidance in orthodontics is highly recommended and easier to establish than group function. A group function is acceptable, but the ideal posterior teeth positioning for this is even more critical. When the canines are periodontally compromised, a group function should be established. Atypical cases of congenitally absent upper lateral incisors, extraction of compromised central lower incisors, or any other case where the premolars are going to replace the canines, should indicate a group function on both sides to prevent future development of traumatic occlusion on the premolars. These teeth are not large enough to support the lateral disclusion forces alone, whereas teeth in group function present as good a periodontal condition as those teeth in canine-guided occlusions.

Every effort to finish with the ideal static and functional occlusion should be made with orthodontic mechanotherapy. The use of Class-II mechanics, with either extraoral anchorage or Class-II elastics, to correct minor anteroposterior shifts of the mandible from CR is recommended. Although advocated, obtaining this ideal finish is mechanically very difficult, and consequently the use of the occlusal adjustment procedure is indicated as an adjunct for the orthodontist to incorporate these details.

Occlusal Adjustment in Orthodontics

Occlusal adjustment is a very exacting procedure that has to be performed judiciously. The neophyte should always have his or her cases mounted on an articulator, adjust them, and then perform the procedure intraorally. A clinician experienced in the procedure is able, in a well treated case, to determine if the adjustment can be undertaken through an intraoral examination. However, cases where the end result of the equilibration cannot be accurately forecasted should be mounted and adjusted first on an articulator. In orthodontics, occlusal adjustment procedure is easier in finished cases, compared with prosthodontic cases, if attention has been given to finishing with the mandible in CR, and with the other gnathologic objectives. If some discrepancies are still present, they are only minor and can easily be eliminated.

Indications for Occlusal Adjustment in Orthodontics

Although occlusal adjustment is recommended in most orthodontic cases to refine the interocclusal relations and distribute the masticatory forces among all the posterior teeth, there are some situations that most often require its use. These are adult or surgical cases or those with mutilations, asymmetric extractions, Bolton discrepancy, irregular restorations, or abnormal extraction protocols. The procedure is applicable in cases with a healthy dentition if one considers that in most cases the orthodontic therapy leaves the teeth in positions other than where they have been worn.

Although no scientific evidence is given, it is the opinion of many recognized authorities that the presence of prematurities and interferences in finished orthodontic cases has a greater potential to cause relapse, that these cases require a longer retention period, and that occlusal adjustment after orthodontic treatment may reduce the need for retainers and the tendency to relapse.

Timing of the Equilibration

The best time to perform occlusal adjustment is at the end of active treatment. There are no rigid rules regarding the timing of the procedure. It is recommended that the larger interferences be taken out immediately after bracket removal because they may cause relapse of the corrected teeth positioning. One month later, during the retention period, when some settling of the occlusion has occurred, a refinement of the equilibration should be conducted. When the patient comes for the next retention visit, usually after 6 months, the occlusion should be checked again, and if there are still any interferences, these should be eliminated. These are only basic guidelines. Sometimes, when near completion of orthodontic treatment, some tooth reshaping can be performed to eliminate any premature contact in CR or any interference during functional mandibular movements, as long as tooth positioning is satisfactory. In some cases, the time necessary to eliminate these interferences through orthodontic tooth movement would be very long, and there might be too many side effects. In these situations, occlusal adjustment is indicated before bracket removal. There are still other occasions in which some tooth reshaping has to be undertaken during treatment to facilitate tooth movement, interocclusal relations, and patient comfort, as in molar uprighting.

There is some controversy regarding who should perform the equilibration. Some orthodontists prefer to refer patients to a prosthodontist experienced with the procedure, whereas others believe that the occlusal adjustment should be performed by the orthodontist himself, instead of referring the patients to a specialist. As mentioned earlier, if the mechanotherapy is conducted to incorporate the functional objectives in the orthodontic treatment, there will be only minor prematurities in CR and interferences during function that can easily be eliminated by the orthodontist experienced with the procedure. The contemporary orthodontist should not only treat the morphologic, but the functional malocclusion as well.

Common Interference Sites in Orthodontic Cases

In orthodontic cases, there are some factors that usually tend to present interferences during the finishing stages. The most common are insufficient lingual crown torque of the upper second molars; accentuated lingual crown torque of the lower second molars; incorrect anteroposterior relation between the maxilla and the mandible; and incoordination of the upper and lower arch widths. These factors can induce interferences in the balancing side. During treatment, these potential interference factors should be corrected by orthodontic mechanotherapy.

Lower Incisor Extraction and Functional Occlusion

The decision to treat a borderline case with a lower incisor extraction requires careful consideration of the resulting functional occlusion. Extraction of a lower incisor is indicated mostly in cases of a severe Bolton discrepancy, compromised lower incisor, or when minimum modification of the profile is required. Cases in which there is a severe Bolton discrepancy, with disproportionately larger lower anterior teeth than upper anterior teeth, usually present a good relation of these teeth at the end of treatment, when one lower incisor is extracted. On the other hand, if the discrepancy is not severe enough, the anterior guidance will be compromised because the upper anterior teeth curvature radius will be disproportionately larger than the lower anterior teeth curvature radius as long as there is a normal buccal intercuspation. The anteroposterior distance of the lower to the upper anterior teeth will be increased, and consequently the anterior teeth will not be able to disclude the posterior teeth on the beginning of protrusion. As a result, many interferences on posterior teeth may develop. Cuspid guidance will also be compromised, because the ideal relation of 0.0005 inch between these teeth will not be established. Moreover, there will be a tendency for relapse of the overbite and overjet.

Occlusal Adjustment Technique and Rules

A brief description of the occlusal adjustment rules is provided. For a more detailed explanation, the reader is referred to Guichet.

The recommended occlusal adjustment technique starts with the equilibration of the mandible in CR. To perform the procedure, the patient has to be in a reclined position, with the chin pointing slightly upward. This position helps guide the mandible into CR because of the effects of gravity as well as the stretching of the retrusive musculature as the patient positions his or her chin upward. A dental assistant has to position the articulating paper between the teeth to identify the premature contacts, as the professional manipulates the mandible to CR bilaterally. Once the premature contacts are identified, grinding is performed on the inclines to alter or reshape all inclines into either cusp tips or flat surfaces. Contacts of cusp tips to flat surfaces direct the occlusal forces through the long axes of the teeth. As the initial premature contacts are eliminated, more teeth will come into contact and have to be adjusted by the same technique, until all posterior teeth make contact evenly.

Once the mandible is stable in CR, the functional excursions can be equilibrated, starting with the balancing sides. The patient should be assisted to perform the lateral excursions to overcome neuromuscular protection. The centric stop cusp tips and their inner inclines are the structures that usually present interferences. When there is an interference between opposing cusp inclines, grinding should be distributed among them. If the interference is between a cusp tip and a cusp incline, the incline should be ground. If the contact occurs between two centric stop cusp tips, the least stable in centric should be ground.

After eliminating the interferences on the balancing sides, the working sides are checked. Independent of the interference spot, the sites to be ground are the tips or inclines of the buccal upper or lingual lower cusps (guide cusps).

The last step consists of equilibrating the teeth in protrusion. Despite the presence of an anterior guidance, interferences on the posterior teeth usually take place between mesial inclines of the lower cusps and distal inclines of the upper cusps. In the situation, the inclines of the guide cusps should be ground. Finally, if there is an interference of an anterior tooth preventing the even contact of all anterior teeth during protrusion, the lower interfering tooth has to be ground if it presents prematurity in CR as well. When the interfering tooth has no contact in CR, the palatal surface of the opposing contacting tooth has to be ground. In rare occasions, the incisal edges have to be reshaped to distribute the forces among the anterior teeth. Briefly stated, the procedure is complete when all posterior teeth present effective occlusal contacts with the mandible in CR and anterior guidance is established.

General Considerations

To provide good orthodontic results for patients, the orthodontist has to incorporate the ideal static and functional characteristics in his or her cases. This chapter describes the functional objectives and how to incorporate them by diagnosing and monitoring cases throughout treatment in CR. Following these guidelines, if a case presents any small discrepancy between CR and centric occlusion, or any interferences during functional movements at the end of treatment, occlusal adjustment can help eliminate them. This is an approach that can be successfully applied in most patients.

Figure 528

Bilateral manipulation of the mandible into centric relation (CR). The patient is in a reclined position, with the chin pointing slightly upward. This position helps guide the mandible into CR because of the effects of gravity and the stretching of the retrusive musculature as the patient positions his or her chin upward. The four fingers of each hand are placed along the lower border of the mandible. The thumbs are positioned over the symphysis of the chin. (Courtesy of Drs. Janson, Martins, Henriques, de Freitas, Pinzan, and de Almeida of the University of São Paulo, Bauru Dental School, Brazil.)

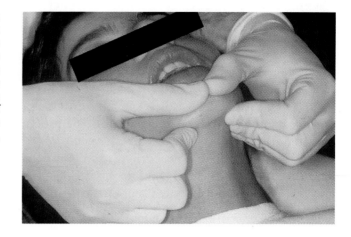

Figures 529–535

Ideal static and functional occlusion in a nonextraction orthodontic case. Figure 529: Frontal view—notice the upper and lower canine positioning to provide disclusion during lateral mandibular movements. Figures 530, 531: Lateral views depicting the correct morphologic buccal intercuspation, with the mandible in centric relation. Figures 532, 533: Disclusion of all posterior teeth provided by the canines on both sides. Figure 534: Disclusion of all posterior teeth provided by the anterior teeth during protrusion. Figure 535: Anterior guidance—there should be no effective contact of the anterior teeth. In centric relation occlusion, there should be a 0.0005-inch clearance between the upper and lower anterior teeth. (Courtesy of Drs. Janson, Martins, Henriques, de Freitas, Pinzan, and de Almeida of the University of São Paulo, Bauru Dental School, Brazil.)

Figure 529

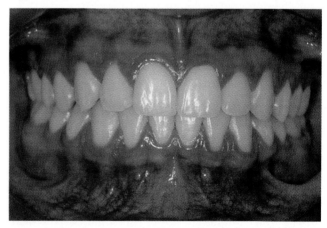

Figure 530

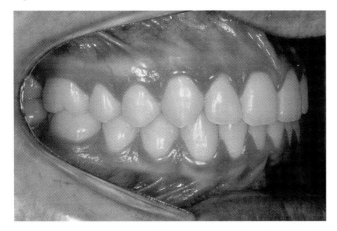

Figure 531

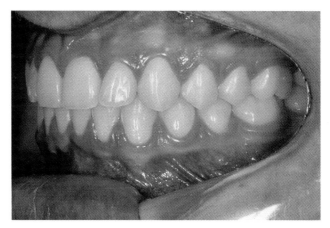

Figure 532

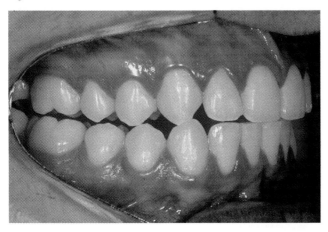

Figure 533

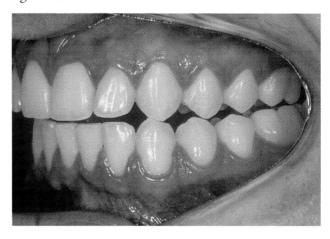

Figure 534

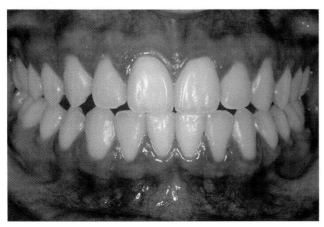

Figure 535

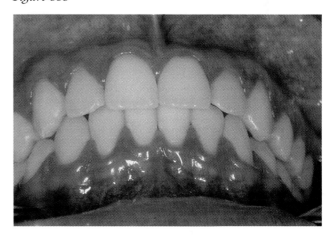

Figures 536–539

Figure 536: Lateral view of a nonextraction finished orthodontic case with the mandible in centric occlusion. Figure 537: Lateral view of the same case, with the mandible in centric relation (CR). Notice the small anteroposterior difference between the upper and lower posterior teeth compared with Figure 536. It is accepted that a well treated, equilibratable orthodontic case should present only minor anteroposterior discrepancies from CR, such as this. Figure 538: Anterior teeth relationship in centric occlusion. Figure 539: Anterior teeth relationship in CR. Notice the small overjet resulting from the discrepancy between centric occlusion and CR. (Courtesy of Drs. Janson, Martins, Henriques, de Freitas, Pinzan, and de Almeida of the University of São Paulo, Bauru Dental School, Brazil.)

Figure 536

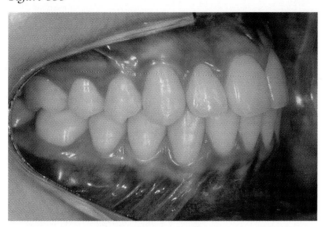

Figure 537

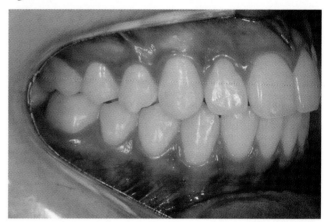

Figure 538

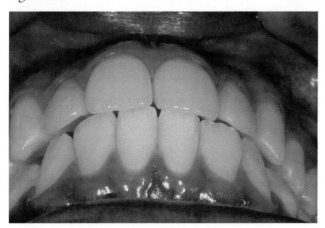

Figure 539

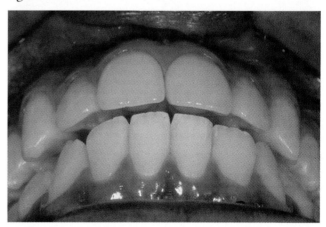

Figures 540–542

Figures 540, 541: Premature contact points that deviate the mandible from centric relation. Figure 542: Grinding of the premature contact point between the buccal cusp tip of the lower first left premolar and the incline of the upper first left premolar palatal cusp. According to Guichet's occlusal adjustment rules, when this type of contact occurs, the incline should be ground flat to direct the occlusal force through the long axis of the tooth. The illustration depicts the grinding being performed with a slow-speed, inverted-cone diamond stone. (Courtesy of Drs. Janson, Martins, Henriques, de Freitas, Pinzan, and de Almeida of the University of São Paulo, Bauru Dental School, Brazil.)

Figure 540

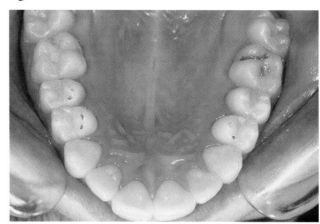

Figure 541

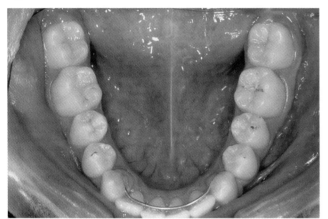

Figure 542

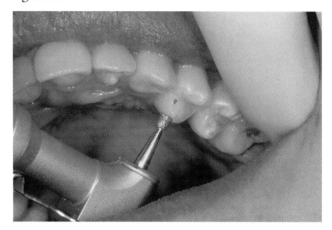

Figures 543–545

Figure 543: Mirror view of the interference between the inner incline of the upper right second molar mesiopalatal cusp and the inner incline of the lower right second molar distobuccal cusp on the right balancing side. Notice that the canines on the left working side cannot establish contact because of this interference. Figure 544: When there is an interference between the inner inclines on the balancing side, the grinding should be distributed among both inclines. This is an illustration of grinding performed on the inner incline of the mesiopalatal cusp of the upper right second molar. This type of interference presents with a marking with a streak characteristic, extending from the centric relation contact. Figure 545: After eliminating the interference, the left canines can disclude the posterior teeth. This case presented no interferences on the working side. (Courtesy of Drs. Janson, Martins, Henriques, de Freitas, Pinzan, and de Almeida of the University of São Paulo, Bauru Dental School, Brazil.)

Figure 543

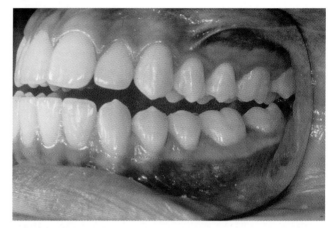

Figure 544

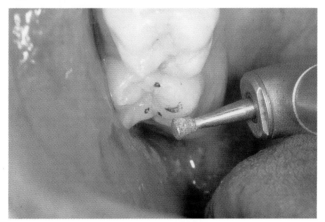

Figure 545

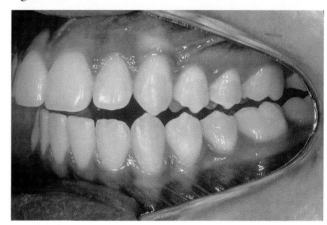

Figures 546, 547

Figure 546: Interferences in protrusion. The upper left central incisor is not establishing contact with the lower incisors because there is an interference of the upper right central incisor. Figure 547: Judicious grinding of the upper right central incisor distal edge allowed the upper left central incisor to establish contact (the right central incisor presented a slight distal tipping that should have been corrected by orthodontic mechanotherapy). (Courtesy of Drs. Janson, Martins, Henriques, de Freitas, Pinzan, and de Almeida of the University of São Paulo, Bauru Dental School, Brazil.)

Figure 546

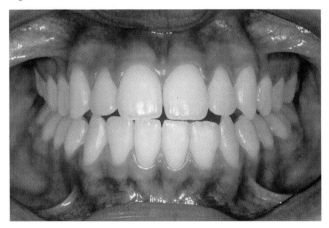

Figure 547

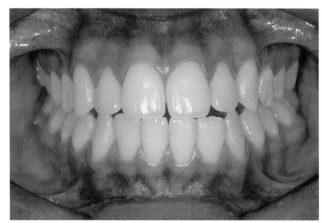

Figures 548, 549

Figure 548: Establishment of anterior guidance after completion of the occlusal adjustment in centric relation (CR). Despite providing canine guidance with disclusion of the posterior teeth, the right canines' positioning is less than ideal in this case. Ideally, there should be less overbite and the upper canine tip should be closer to the lower canine buccal surface. Compare with Figure 535. Figure 549: Test of the 0.0005-inch clearance in the anterior region with a shimstock. The shimstock is held in CR by the anterior teeth, but can slip through under traction. (Courtesy of Drs. Janson, Martins, Henriques, de Freitas, Pinzan, and de Almeida of the University of São Paulo, Bauru Dental School, Brazil.)

Figure 548

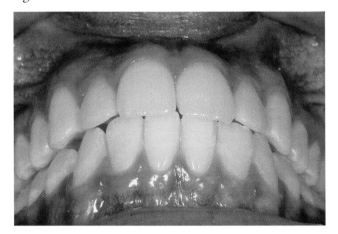

Figure 549

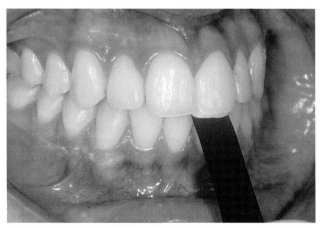

Frontal and lateral views of the case after completion of the occlusal adjustment. The mandible is now in centric relation. (Courtesy of Drs. Janson, Martins, Henriques, de Freitas, Pinzan, and de Almeida of the University of São Paulo, Bauru Dental School, Brazil.)

Figure 550

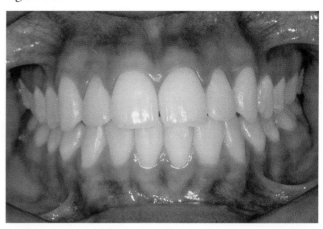

Figure 551

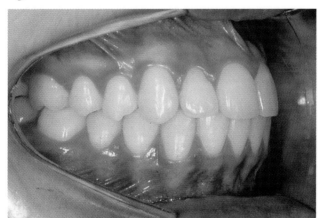

Figure 552

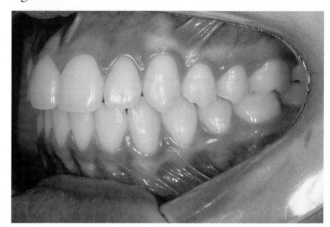

Retention Facts and Protocol

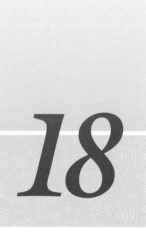

Over the past 30 years, a number of studies have dealt with the stability of orthodontic treatment after the retention phase. Two thirds of 65 patients examined 10 years postretention, previously treated in the permanent dentition stage with first bicuspid extractions and traditional edgewise mechanics, had unsatisfactory lower anterior alignment after retention. In a follow-up study 20 years postretention, only 10% of the cases were judged to have clinically acceptable mandibular alignment (compared with 30% at the 10-year phase). The teeth of patients who had undergone serial extraction plus comprehensive treatment and retention were no better aligned postretention than were those in late extraction cases. There is considerable long-term stability for most cases of mild to moderate malocclusions treated without extractions. Arch length shows significant reduction postretention, similar to that of untreated normal subjects and extraction cases (2–2.5 mm). The patient's pretreatment arch form appeared to be the best guide to future arch form stability, but minimizing treatment change was no guarantee of postretention stability (Figures 553, 554).

In untreated normal subjects, we see decreases in arch length and intercuspid width; minimal overall changes in intermolar width, overjet, and overbite; and increases in incisor irregularity. When comparing mandibular anterior alignment in this sample to that reported in most of the articles reviewed, the prolonged retention time may be an important factor. It also appears that arch expansion in the premolar regions, particularly in the maxillary arch, is relatively stable. Furthermore, no associations or predictors of clinical value are known with regard to assessing stability or relapse. Maturational changes in the permanent dentition of a sample of untreated normal subjects appear, in general, to be similar in nature to those of a postretention sample of treated cases. Orthodontic therapy may temporarily alter the course of the continuous physiologic changes and, possibly, for a time, even reverse them; however, after mechanotherapy and the period of retention restraint, the developmental maturation process resumes.

There is little doubt that relapse of orthodontically rotated teeth is primarily due to the displaced supraalveolar connective tissue fibers. A simple surgical method of severing all supracrestal fibrous attachment (circumferential supracrestal fiberotomy) to a rotated tooth has been shown significantly to alleviate relapse after rotation, with no apparent damage to the supporting structures of the teeth.

Teeth that are orthodontically moved together after extraction of an adjacent tooth do not move through the gingival tissue but appear to push the gingiva ahead to create a fold of epithelial and connective tissues. After the final closure of an extraction site, this excess gingival tissue appears in papillary form buccally and lingually between the approximated teeth. By surgically removing the excess gingiva between properly approximated teeth, relapse can be alleviated.

Instability should be assumed because it is the more likely pattern. Permanent retention, either with fixed or removable retainers, seems to be the logical answer (see Figure 553). Patients and parents should be informed of the risk of relapse and the limitations of treatment before treatment begins, and patients should expect to remain in retention long term, with monitoring continuing throughout the patient's adult life.

In most cases, the maxillary second molars are not bonded during treatment. In most instances, provided that the mandibular second molars are in good position, the pressure of the buccinator muscles and normal eruption will move the maxillary second molars into proper position.

Figure 553

A patient's beautiful smile needs to be retained throughout life. Just as we keep coloring our hair, permanent retention for 2 or 3 nights a week would maintain a youthful smile, as the process of aging slowly sets in.

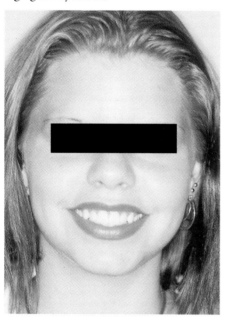

Figure 554

Permanent (lifetime) retention is recommended. The patient wears the upper/lower Essix removable retainers full time for 12 months. After the first year, the upper is worn during sleeping hours and the lower during the day. The patient wears the retainers 3 nights a week permanently to maintain the youthful smile and counteract changes due to the aging process.

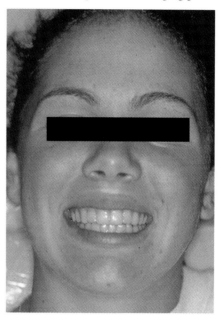

Cosmetic Dentistry and Periodontics

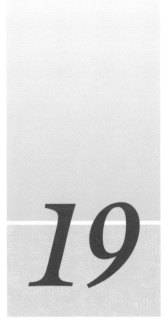

19

An attractive smile has always been the focal point of improving a person's esthetic appearance and thus self-esteem. It is the contrasts of shape, color, line, and texture that enable us to differentiate one tooth from another, the teeth from the gums, and the smile from the face. We perceive an ideal smile as bright, vigorous, and youthful, regardless of age. From a cultural standpoint, a prominent smile with bright teeth is synonymous with youth and dynamism. This ideal smile is based on an intact and well aligned, harmonious dentition (Figures 555–601).

A smile is formed within the border of the lips. There are distinct elements contributing to a smile, including the incisal edges, the gingival embrasures, the gingival height of contour, and the interproximal contact areas. Tooth color and texture are two elements that require particular attention in a complete esthetic composite. Last, the gingival tissues and the dark space and opposing dentition all combine to form the perfect smile.

Ideally, a smile line is in harmony with the lower lip and parallel to the interpupillary axis. The edges of the teeth may approach or even lightly touch the lower lip. This is a reference point that helps establish correct and pleasing tooth length. The gingival height of contour ideally follows the contour of the upper lip and may approach, touch, or be slightly hidden beneath it.

Upper lip support is controlled to a certain extent by the position of the maxillary teeth. The gingival two thirds rather than the incisal one third of the maxillary central incisors contribute the main support of the lip. When the "F" or "V" consonant sounds are pronounced, the incisal edges should make a definite contact at the inner vermilion border of the lower lip.

Gingival asymmetry of the maxillary central incisors requires special attention. Incisal and gingival embrasures are key elements that begin to define the individual identity of a tooth within a smile. Variations in embrasure form contribute to the notion of feminine- or masculine-looking smiles. Deep, round embrasures appear more youthful and feminine, whereas narrow, short embrasures present a harsher, worn look, and typify masculine-looking teeth. In general, women show almost twice as much tooth as men. Youth is expressed with prominent and well developed central incisors, well defined incisal embrasures, and a convex or "gull wing" smile line.

Interproximal contact areas define the individuality of each tooth within the same smile. The dominance of the central incisors over the supporting elements is clear. The two centrals are so dominant, they may take up 30% to 50% of the total viewing area of a smile.

Gingival tissues are most pleasing when seen as papillae with a minimal show of keratinized and, especially, mucosal tissue. The "gummy smile" is often encountered in patients who have short lip lines or where more than 3 mm of gingiva in the maxillary anterior region is displayed during a relaxed smile. Proper incisal position must first be evaluated in relation to the lips, then an average tooth length of pleasing proportion should be visualized from this incisal edge.

More often than not, there is a need for "feminizing" the incisal edges after orthodontic correction in cases of malocclusion. In fact, probably all orthodontic cases may benefit from recontouring of the incisal edges.

Sometimes, when the crown lengths of the right and left central and lateral incisors are compared, there is a significant difference in the length of the teeth. This unesthetic oblique incisal plane is caused by a combination of asymmetric wear of the incisors and uneven eruption of the anterior teeth. Treatment requires a combination of orthodontics to level the gingival margins and restorative dentistry to recreate symmetric lengths of the right and left central and lateral incisors.

Abnormalities in tooth size and shape can detract from the final esthetic outcome of orthodontic treatment. In many cases, these unesthetic situations can be improved through a coordinated teamwork approach of orthodontics, periodontics, and restorative dentistry. It is important, therefore, to evaluate four aspects of the maxillary anterior teeth and gingiva: crown length, crown width, crown form, and gingival form.

Prosthodontists rely on a proportion of 17:1 for the relation between the central and lateral incisors. When recontouring the canines, it is important to evaluate the lateral excursive contacts to ensure that canine contact will be preserved in the lateral working relation.

Clinicians must look not only at alignment, but evaluate crown length, crown width, crown form, and gingival form when evaluating the esthetics of the maxillary anterior teeth. Small adjustments in tooth morphology, position, and gingival form can enhance the esthetic appearance of future anterior restorative treatment and help to produce a more beautiful smile.

After orthodontics, cosmetic dentistry can create a beautiful smile with a variety of techniques and materials, often in just one or two appointments. A new look can be achieved just by whitening the teeth, or it can involve more complex treatments such as bonding, laminates, crowns, bridges, or implants.

For years, covering exposed roots with soft tissue grafting has been the ultimate goal in periodontal mucogingival surgery. Today, that goal has been largely met with the use of various techniques. The larger arena of esthetic enhancement now dominates our thought processes in dentistry. "Periodontal plastic surgery" is the term used to describe surgical procedures performed to correct or eliminate anatomic, developmental, or traumatic deformities of the gingiva and alveolar mucosa. These procedures would also include treatment of marginal tissue recession, excessive gingival margins, and localized alveolar ridge deficiency, as well as exposure of unerupted teeth for orthodontic treatment.

Throughout history, smiles have been the ultimate form of communication. Today, orthodontists, cosmetic dentists, and periodontists can make perfect smiles easier and better than ever.

Figures 555–558

Bonding, a completely painless process that can be done in just one visit, can mask stains and cover any flaws through the placement of a thin plastic coating on the front surface of the teeth. This teenager did not like the shape of and the white spots on her four front teeth. After priming the tooth surface, a putty-like bonding material is applied and then sculpted, shaped, and colored to perfect a smile. A high-intensity light or laser causes the plastic to harden, after which it is smoothed and polished. Bonding can lighten teeth, close gaps, and even alter malformed teeth. It can be used to change the shape or color of a single tooth or, in some cases, revitalize an entire smile. (Courtesy of Dr. Lorin Berland.)

Figure 555

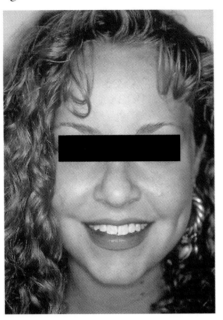

Figure 556

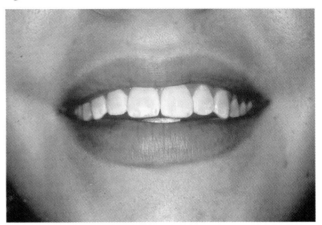

Figure 557

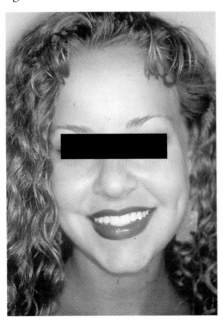

Figure 558

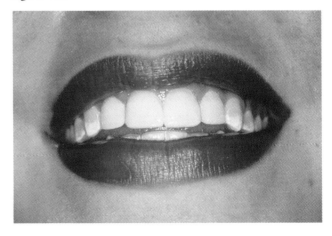

This young woman had uneven spaces that put a shadow on her smile. Bonding of her six front teeth whitened and widened her teeth to give her a big, beautiful smile. (Courtesy of Dr. Lorin Berland.)

Figure 559

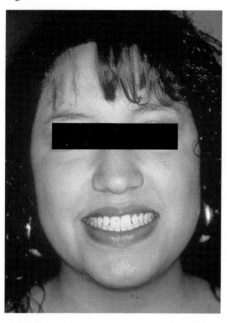

Figure 560

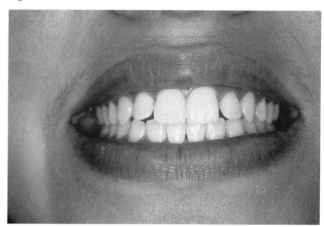

Figure 561

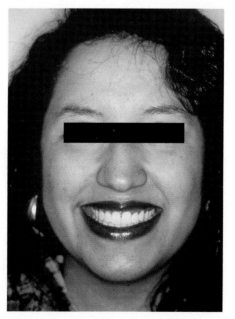

Figure 562

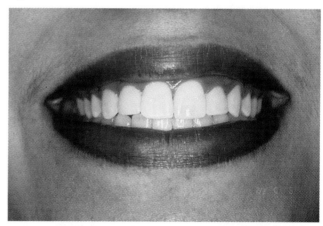

Figures 563, 564

Some smile rehabilitations are beyond the scope of bonding. In these cases, porcelain veneers are indicated for their strength and durability. Procelain is best for correcting major functional or structural problems with individual or missing teeth. This young woman is missing a front tooth that has been replaced temporarily. Her lower teeth are professionally whitened, and 10 custom-made, ultrathin porcelain veneers are created to replace the missing tooth and beautify her smile. This new look is typically accomplished in two visits. The teeth are prepared and impressions are taken at the first appointment. The veneers are fabricated in the laboratory and bonded to the teeth at the next appointment. (Courtesy of Dr. Lorin Berland.)

Figure 563

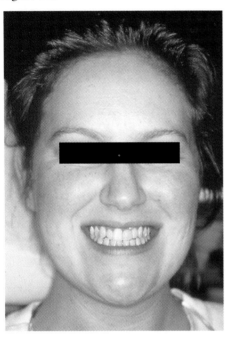

Figure 564

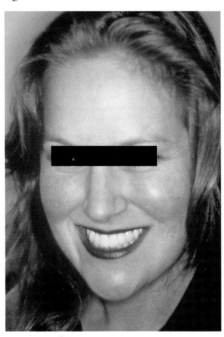

Figures 565, 566

The end result of an orthodontically treated occlusion needs to take into consideration the dental condition of the patient. This patient had flat proximal contacts between the first molars and the second premolars, resulting in potential further decay in those sites. Because this patient was treated with extraction of the upper second premolars for orthodontic reasons, note that the final contacts of the first premolars to the first molars are point contacts instead of flat surfaces. The molars were deliberately finished slightly rotated to obtain these contacts so that the patient would have an easier time flossing and keeping that area clean. (Courtesy of Dr. Lorin Berland.)

Figure 565

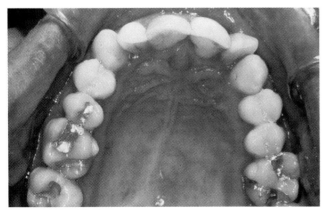

Figure 566

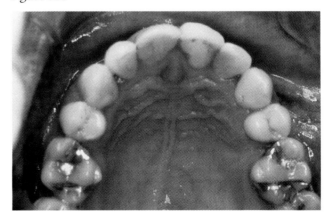

Figures 567, 568

Sometimes cosmetic bonding is not enough truly to enhance the patient's final smile outline. Periodontal plastic surgery is often indicated to create a beautiful smile. This patient needed such plastic gum recontouring on the upper lateral incisors. The patient refused such treatment, even though it would have further accentuated her smile.

Figure 567

Figure 568

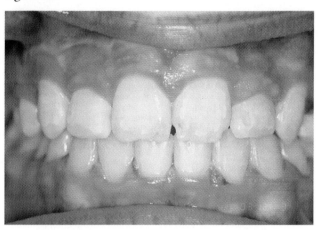

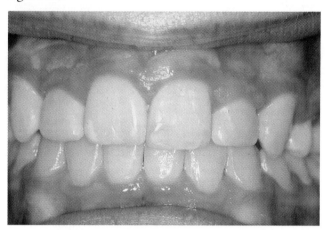

Figures 569–574

Excessive gingival display is a condition resulting from excessive exposure of maxillary gingiva during smiling, commonly called gummy smile or high lip line. This condition may be caused by a skeletal deformity, a soft tissue deformity, or a combination of the two. Another cause is short clinical crowns due to incomplete exposure of the anatomic crowns. If short clinical crowns result in a gummy smile, gingival contouring may be accomplished to achieve the desired esthetic result. The gummy smile can be managed to create proper clinical crown length and achieve pleasing gingival contours. Diagnosis of this problem can be made by the orthodontist early in treatment. Evaluation of the smile line, lip line, and tooth length can help differentiate between excessive gingival display due to vertical maxillary excess or insufficient crown length. Furthermore, the establishment of the marginal tissue at the level of the cement–enamel junction enhances esthetics and creates a situation that gives the orthodontist a larger "comfort zone" when treating periodontally involved cases. Periodontal plastic surgery involves a flap in the area of interest, and bone and soft tissue recontouring to enhance the gingival outline with the tooth incisal edge outlines. The benefits of such a procedure are obvious, as shown on the patient's postsurgical outline.

Figure 569

Figure 570

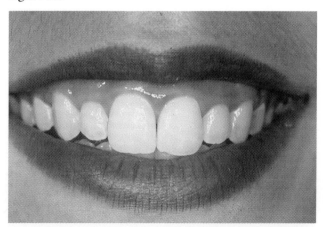

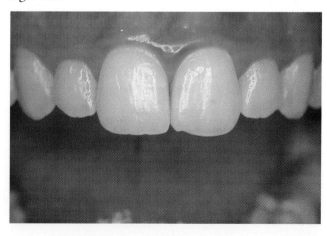

Figure 571

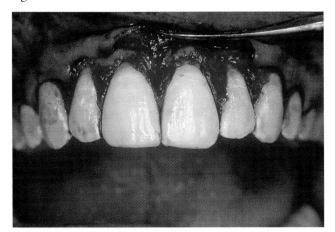

Figure 572

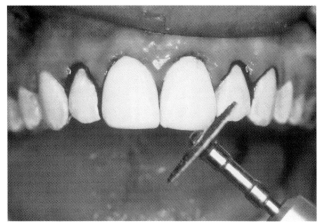

Figure 573

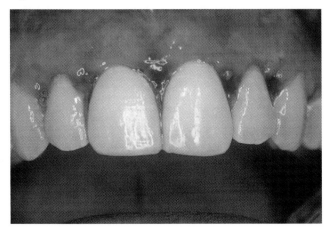

Figure 574

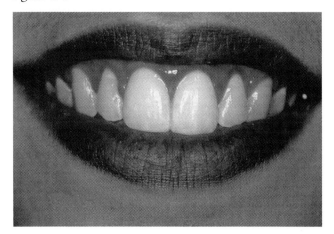

Successful root coverage techniques can aid in the treatment of inadequately attached gingiva as well as root sensitivity and unesthetic appearance. Root coverage techniques for treatment of canine marginal tissue recession in the past have been relatively unpredictable procedures. Soft tissue grafting was done primarily to increase the band on attached gingiva. In 1982, a preditable technique was described for covering roots using the free gingival graft after citric acid root conditioning. In 1985, the subepithelial connective tissue graft for improved esthetics in root coverage grafting was introduced. Since then, it has proved especially useful in the treatment of gingival recession. (Courtesy of Dr. Elizabeth Jaynes.)

Figure 575

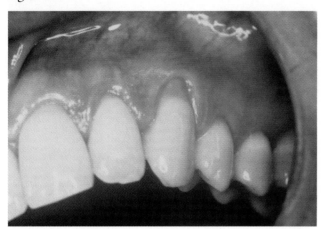

Figure 576

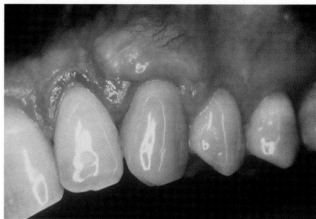

Figure 577

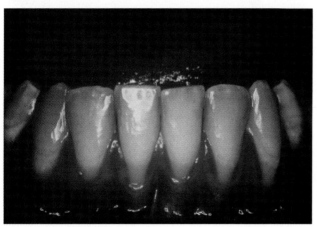

Figure 578

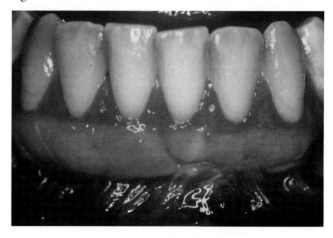

Figures 579–601

This patient was given a treatment time estimate of 2 to 3 years of therapy and extraction of four premolars with the old, square brackets and stainless steel mechanics. She was treated nonextraction with tooth recontouring in the upper arch and an incisor extraction in the lower arch, the new triangular brackets, and one set of superelastic wires in just 8 months! The radiographs (root position, parallelism, and inclination) demonstrate the excellence of the treatment result. If cases like this one can be finished in such a short period of time, then the future of orthodontics is indeed very bright for patients and doctors alike.

Figure 579

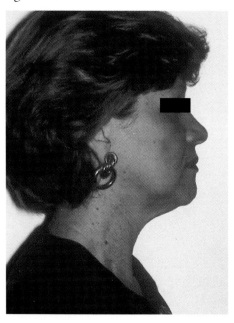

Figure 580

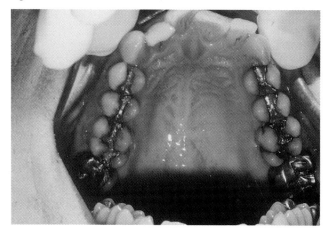

Figure 581

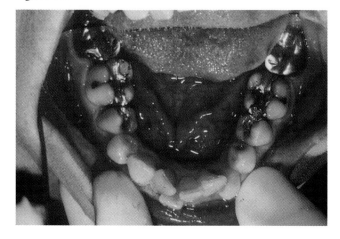

Figure 582

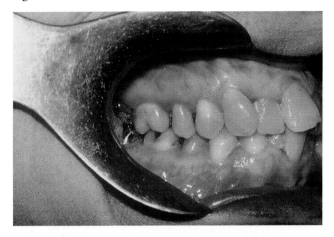

Figure 583

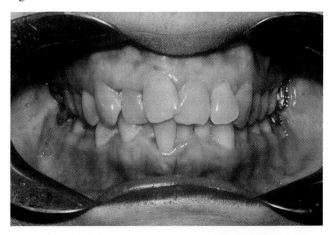

Figure 584

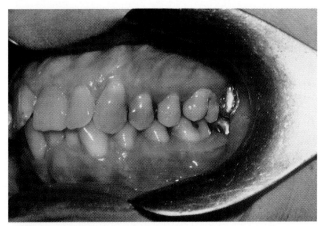

Figure 585

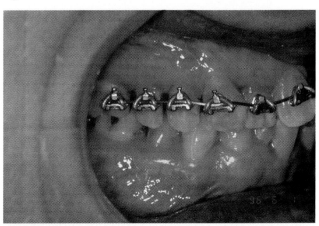

Figure 586

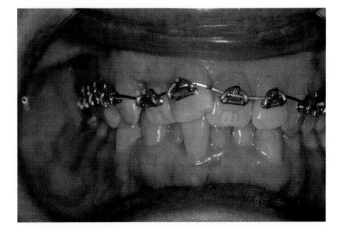

Figure 587

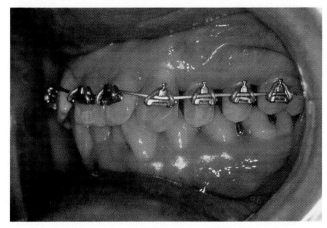

Figure 588

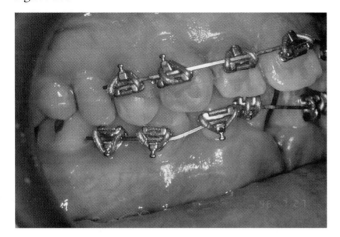

Figure 589

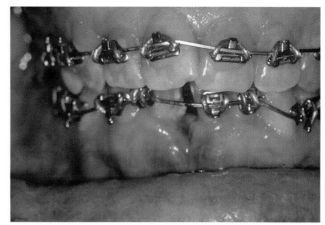

Figure 590

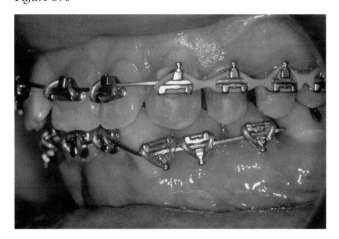

Figure 591

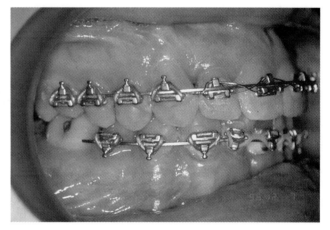

Figure 592

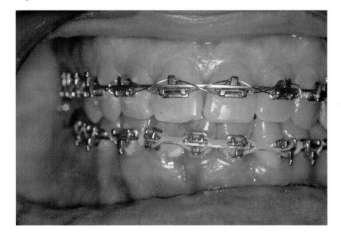

Figure 593

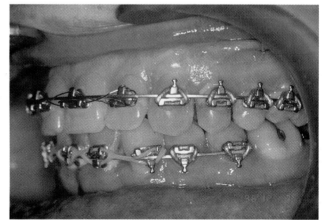

Figure 594

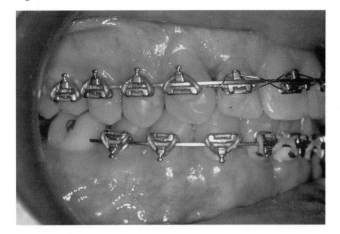

Figure 595

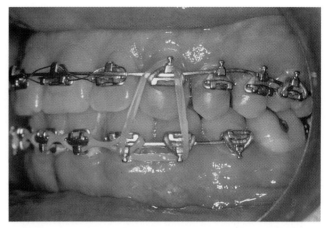

Figure 596

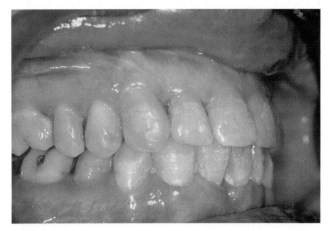

Figure 597

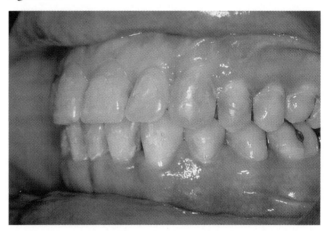

Figure 598

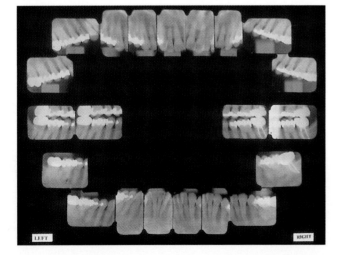

Figure 599

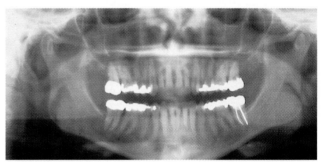

Figure 600

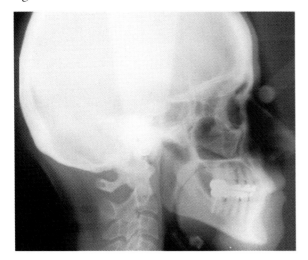

Figure 601

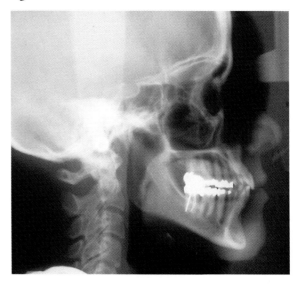

The future is bright!

Bibliography

Ackerman JL, Proffit WR: Communication in orthodontic treatment planning: bioethical and informed consent issues. Angle Orthod 65:253–262, 1995.

Ades R, Joondeph D, Little R, Chapko M. A long term study of the relationship of third molars to changes in the mandibular dental arch. Am J Orthod Dentofacial Orthop 97:323–335, 1990.

Alexander RG: The vari-simplex discipline: Part 4. countdown to retention. J Clin Orthod 9:619–625, 1983.

Alexander RG: *The Alexander Discipline: Contemporary Concepts and Philosophies.* Glendora, CA: Ormco Co., 1986.

Alexander RG: Countdown to retention. J Clin Orthod 21:526–529, 1987.

Alexander SA: Levels of root resorption associated with continuous arch and sectional arch mechanics. Am J Orthod Dentofacial Orthop 110:321–324, 1996.

Allen EP: Use of mucogingival surgical procedures to enhance esthetics. Dent Clin North Am 32:307–330, 1988.

American Academy of Craniomandibular Disorders: *Craniomandibular Disorders: Guidelines for Evaluation, Diagnosis and Management.* McNeill D, ed. Chicago: Quintessence Publishing, 1988.

American Academy of Craniomandibular Disorders: *Craniomandibular Disorders: Guidelines for Evaluation, Diagnosis and Management.* 2nd ed. McNeill C, ed. Chicago: Quintessence Publishing, 1990.

American Association of Orthodontists: Oral habits: Non-nutritive sucking and tongue thrusting. Orthodontic Dialogue 4:2–3, 1991.

Andreasen GF, Hilleman TB: An evaluation of 55 cobalt substituted nitinol wire for use in orthodontics. J Am Dent Assoc 82:1373–1375, 1972.

Andreasen GF, Morrow RD: Laboratory and clinical analyses of nitinol wire. Am J Orthod 73:142–151, 1978.

Andreasen GF, Quevado FR: Evaluation of the friction forces in the 0.022″ × 0.028″ edgewise bracket in vitro. J Biomech 3:151–160, 1970.

Andrews LA: The six keys to normal occlusion. Am J Orthod 62:296–309, 1972.

Andrews LF: The straight-wire appliance: origin, controversy, commentary. J Clin Orthod 10(2):99–114, 1976.

Andrews LF: *Straight Wire: Concept and Appliances.* San Diego, CA: L.A. Wells Co., 1989.

Angolkar PV, et al: Evaluation of friction between ceramic brackets and orthodontic wires of four alloys. Am J Orthod 98:499–506, 1990.

Argyropoulos E, Payne G: Technique for improving orthodontic results in the treatment of

missing maxillary incisors: a case report with literature review. Am J Orthod Dentofacial Orthop 94:150–165, 1988.

Arnett GW: Excellent treatment results using ideal orthodontic/orthognathic treatment planning. Summarized by Nichols LO. Pacific Coast Society of Orthodontists Bulletin 37–39, 1991.

Artun J: Long-term periodontal response to orthodontic treatment: summary by Hawley B. Pacific Coast Society of Orthodontists Bulletin, Spring, 42–43, 1991.

Arvystas MG: Nonextraction treatment of severe class II, division 2 malocclusions. Am J Orthod Dentofacial Orthop 99:74–84, 1991.

Baker KL, et al: Frictional changes in force values caused by saliva substitution. Am J Orthod 91:316–320, 1987.

Bandeen RL, Timm TA: Temporomandibular joint dysfunction: report of a case. Am J Orthod Dentofacial Orthop 87:275–279, 1985.

Barrett R, et al: Biodegradation of orthodontic appliances: Part I. biodegradation of nickel and chromium in vitro. Am J Orthod Dentofacial Orthop 103:8–14, 1993.

Bass J, et al: Nickel hypersensibility in the orthodontic patient. Am J Orthod Dentofacial Orthop 103:280–285, 1993.

Bass NM: The aesthetic analysis of the face. Eur J Orthod 13:343–350, 1991.

Baty D, et al: Force delivery properties of colored elastomeric modules. Am J Orthod Dentofacial Orthop 106:40–46, 1994.

Baumrind S, Korn EL, West EE: Prediction of mandibular rotation: an empirical test of clinician performance. Am J Orthod 86:371–385, 1984.

Baumrind S, et al: Apical root resorption in orthodontically treated adults. Am J Orthod Dentofacial Orthop 110:311–320, 1996.

Beck B, Harris E: Apical root resorption in orthodontically treated subjects: analysis of eclusive and light wire mechanics. Am J Orthod Dentofacial Orthop 105:350–361, 1994.

Becks H: Orthodontic prognosis: evaluation of routine dentomedical examination to determine "good and poor risks." Am J Orthod 25:610–624, 1939.

Bednar JR, Gruendeman GW, Sandrik JL: A comparison study of frictional forces between orthodontic brackets and arch wires. Am J Orthod 100:513–522, 1991.

Bell R, Kiyak HA, Joondeph DR: Perceptions of facial profile and their influence on the decision to undergo orthognathic surgery. Am J Orthod Dentofacial Orthop 88:323, 1985.

Bell WH: *Surgical Correction of Dentofacial Deformities.* Vol II. St. Louis, MO: CV Mosby, 1986.

Bell, WH, et al: Treatment of a class II deep bite by orthodontic and surgical means. Am J Orthod Dentofacial Orthop 85:1–20, 1984.

Bishara S, et al: Biodegration of orthodontic appliances: Part II. changes in the blood level of nickel. Am J Orthod Dentofacial Orthop 103:115–119, 1993.

Bishara S, et al: Longitudinal comparisons of dental arch changes in normal and untreated class II, division 1 subjects and their clinical implications. Am J Orthod Dentofacial Orthop 110:683–689, 1996.

Bishara SE: Impacted maxillary canines: a review. Am J Orthod Dentofacial Orthop 101: 159–171, 1992.

Bishara SE, Hoppens BJ, Jacobsen JR, Kohout FJ: Changes in the molar relationship between the deciduous and permanent dentition: a longitudinal study. Am J Orthod Dentofacial Orthop 93:19–28, 1988.

Bishara SE, Staley RN: Maxillary expansion: clinical implications. Am J Orthod Dentofacial Orthop 91:3–14, 1987.

Bishara SE, Ziaga RR: Functional appliances: a review. Am J Orthod Dentofacial Orthop 95:250–258, 1989.

Björk A: Cranial base development. Am J Orthod 41:198–255, 1955.

Björk A: Variations in the growth pattern of the human mandible: longitudinal radiographic study by the implant method. J Dent Res 42:400–411, 1963.

Björk A, Skiller V: Facial development and tooth eruption: an implant study at the age of puberty. Am J Orthod 62:331–383, 1972.

Björk A, Skiller V: Normal and abnormal growth of the mandible: a synthesis of longitudinal cephalometric implant studies over a period of 25 years. Eur J Orthod 5:1–46, 1983.

Blackwood HO III: Clinical management of the Jasper Jumper. J Clin Orthod 25:755–760, 1991.

Blake M, et al: A radiographic comparison of apical root resorption after orthodontic treatment with the edgewise and Speed appliances. Am J Orthod Dentofacial Orthop 108:76–84, 1995.

Blume DG: A study of occlusal equilibration as it relates to orthodontics. Am J Orthod 44:575–584, 1958.

Boese L: Fiberotomy and reproximation without lower retention, nine years in retrospect: Part I. Angle Orthod 50:88–97, 1980.

Boese L: Fiberotomy and reproximation without lower retention, nine years in retrospect: Part II. Angle Orthod 50:169–178, 1980.

Boyd RL: Can adults with periodontitis be treated orthodontically? Summary by Quinn RS. Pacific Coast Society of Orthodontists Bulletin, Spring, 48–49, 1991.

Boyd RL, Murray P, Robertson PB: Effect from electric toothbrush versus manual toothbrush on periodontal status during orthodontic treatment. Am J Orthod Dentofacial Orthop 96:342–347, 1989.

Boyd R, Rose C: Effect of rotary electric toothbrush versus manual toothbrush on decalcification during orthodontic treatment. An J Orthod Dentofacial Orthop 105:450–456, 1994.

Brezniak N, Wasserstein A: Root resorption after orthodontic treatment: Part 1. literature review. Am J Orthod Dentofacial Orthop 103:62–66, 1993a.

Brezniak N, Wasserstein A: Root resorption after orthodontic treatment: Part 2. literature review. Am J Orthod Dentofacial Orthop 103:138–143, 1993b.

Brin I, Becker A, Zilberman Y: Resorbed lateral incisors adjacent to impacted canines have normal crown size. Am J Orthod Dentofacial Orthop 104:60–66, 1993.

Brodie G: Late growth changes in the human face. Angle Orthod 23:147–157, 1953.

Burke S, et al: Incidence and size of pretreatment overlap and postreatment gingival embrasure space between maxillary central incisors. Am J Orthod Dentofacial Orthop 105:506–511, 1994.

Burstone CJ: The integumental profile. Am J Orthod 44:1–25, 1958.

Burstone CJ: Integumental contour and extension patterns. Angle Orthod 29:93–104, 1959.

Burstone CJ: Variable-modulus orthodontics. Am J Orthod 80:1–16, 1981.

Burstone CJ, Farzin-Nia F: Production of low friction and colored TMA by ion-implantation. J Clin Orthod 29:453–461, 1995.

Burstone CJ, Goldberg AJ: Beta-titanium: a new orthodontic alloy. Am J Orthod 77: 121–132, 1980.

Burstone CJ, Qin B, Morton JY: Chinese NiTi wire: a new orthodontic alloy. Am J Orthod 87:445–452, 1985.

Burstone CR: Deep overbite correction by intrusion. Am J Orthod 72:1–22, 1977.

Buschang PH, LaPalme L, Tanguay R, Demirjian A: The technical reliability of superimposition on cranial base and mandibular structures. Eur J Orthod 8:152–156, 1986.

Buschang PH, Viazis AD, DelaCruz R, Oakes C: Horizontal growth of the soft-tissue nose relative to maxiuary growth. J Clin Orthod 26:111–118, 1992.

Campbell PM: The dilemma of class III treatment. Angle Orthod 53:175–191, 1983.

Cannon J: Head posture: an historical review of the literature. Aust Orthod 9:234–237, 1985.

Cetlin NM, Ten Hoeve A: Nonextraction therapy. J Clin Orthod 17:396–413, 1983.

Chabre C: Vertical control with a headgear–activator combination. J Clin Orthod 24: 618–624, 1990.

Chaconas SJ: A statistical evaluation of nasal growth. Am J Orthod 56:403–414, 1969.

Chang HP: Assessment of anteroposterior jaw relationship. Am J Orthod 92:117–122, 1987.

Chateau M: *Orthopedie Dentofaciale: Bases Fondamentales.* Paris: Julien Prélat, 1975.

Chau LT, et al: Force decay of elastomeric chain: a serial study. Part II. Am J Orthod Dentofacial Orthop 104:373–377, 1993.

Chiappone RC: A gnathologic approach to orthodontic finishing. J Clin Orthod 7:405–417, 1975.

Chiappone RC: Constructing the gnathologic setup and positioner. J Clin Orthod 14: 121–133, 1980.

Chiche G, Pinault A: *Esthetics of Anterior Fixed Prosthodontics.* Chicago: Quintessence Publishing, 1994.

Clements BS: Nasal imbalance and the orthodontic patient. Am J Orthod 55:244–264, 329–352, 477–497, 1969.

Coben SE: The integration of facial skeletal variants. Am J Orthod 41:407–434, 1955.

Coben SE: Basion horizontal coordinate tracing film. J Clin Orthod 13:598–605, 1979.

Cole SC: Natural head position, posture, prognathism. Br J Orthod 15:227–239, 1988.

Cooke MS, Wei SHY: A summary five-factor cephalometric analysis based on natural head posture and the true horizontal. Am J Orthod 93:213–223, 1988.

Crain G, Sheridan JJ: Susceptibility to caries and periodontal disease after posterior air-rotor stripping. J Clin Orthod 24:84–85, 1990.

Creekmore TD: The importance of interbracket width in orthodontic tooth movement. J Clin Orthod 10:530, 1976.

Creekmore TD: Teeth want to be straight. J Clin Orthod 16:745–746, 1982.

Creekmore TD, et al: JCO Roundtable: diagnosis and treatment planning. J Clin Orthod 26:585–606, 1992.

Creekmore TD, Kunik RL: Straight wire: the next generation. Am J Orthod Dentofacial Orthop 104:8, 1993.

Crosby DR, Alexander RG: The occurrence of tooth size discrepancies among different malocclusion groups. Am J Orthod Dentofacial Orthop 95:457–461, 1989.

Dahl EH, Zachrisson BU: Long term evaluation of bonded retainers. J Clin Orthod 25:619–630, 1991.

Daili M, et al.: The orthodontic pain. PhD thesis, research. University of Kuopio, Finland, 1997.

D'Amico A: The canine teeth: the normal functional relation of the natural teeth of man. Journal of the Southern California Dental Association XIXX, 1958.

Davies TM, Shaw WC, Worthington HV, Addy M, Dummer P, Kingdon A: The effect of orthodontic treatment on plaque and gingivitis. Am J Orthod Dentofacial Orthop 99:155–162, 1991.

Dawson PE: *Evaluation, Diagnosis, and Treatment of Occlusal Problems.* St. Louis, MO: CV Mosby, 1974.

de Coster L: The familial line, studies by a new line of reference. Trans Eur Orthod Soc 28:50–55, 1952.

DeFranco DJ, Spiller RE, von Fraunhofer JA: Frictional resistance using Teflon coated ligatures with various bracket–archwire combinations. Angle Orthod 65:63–72, 1995.

De La Cruz A, et al: Long-term changes in arch form after orthodontic treatment and retention. Am J Orthod Dentofacial Orthop 107:518–530, 1995.

Dent B, Blake M, Woodwide DG, Pharoah MJ: A radiographic comparison of apical root resorption after orthodontic treatment with the edgewise and Speed appliances. Am J Orthod Dentofacial Orthop 108:76–84, 1995.

DeShields RW: A study of root resorption in treated class II division I malocclusion. Angle Orthod 39:231–245, 1969.

DeVincenzo JP: Changes in mandibular length before, during and after successful orthopedic correction of class II malocclusions, using a functional appliance. Am J Orthod Dentofacial Orthop 99:241–257, 1991.

Dibbets JMH, van der Weele LT: Extraction, orthodontic treatment, and craniomandibular dysfunction. Am J Orthod Dentofacial Orthop 99:210–219, 1991.

Drobocky OB, Smith RJ: Changes in facial profile during orthodontic treatment with extraction of four basic bicuspids. Am J Orthod Dentofacial Orthop 95:220–230, 1989.

Dougherty HL: The effect of mechanical forces upon the mandibular buccal segments during orthodontic treatment. Part I. Am J Orthod 54:29–49, 1968a.

Dougherty HL. The effect of mechanical forces upon the mandibular buccal segments during orthodontic treatment. Part II. Am J Orthod 54:83–103, 1968b.

Drake SR, et al: Mechanical properties of orthodontic wires in tension, bending and torsion. Am J Orthod 82:206–210, 1982.

Drescher D, Bourauel C, Schumacher H: Frictional forces between brackets and arch wire. Am J Orthod 96:397–404, 1989.

Eales KA, Newton C, Jones ML, Sugar A: The accuracy of computerized prediction of the soft tissue profile: a study of 25 patients treated by means of the LeFort I osteotomy. Int J Adult Orthod Orthognath Surg 9:141–152, 1994.

Edwards J: A surgical procedure to eliminate rotational relapse. Am J Orthod 57:35–46, 1970.

Edwards J: The prevention of relapse in extraction cases. Am J Orthod 60:128–140, 1971.

Edwards J: A long term perspective evaluation of the circumferential supracrestal fibcrotomy in alleviating orthodontic relapse. Am J Orthod 93:380–387, 1988.

Egermark I, Thilander B: Craniomandibular disorders with special reference to orthodontic treatment: an evaluation from childhood to adulthood. Am J Orthod Dentofacial Orthop 101:8–34, 1992.

Egermark-Eriksson, I, et al: The dependence of mandibular dysfunction in children on functional and morphologic malocclusion. Am J Orthod Dentofacial Orthop 83:1974, 1983.

Ehasson LA, Hugoson A, Kurol J, Siwe H: The effects of orthodontic treatment on periodontal tissues in patients with reduced periodontal support. Eur J Orthod 4:1–9, 1982.

Ekstrom C: Facial growth rate and its relation to somatic maturation in healthy children. Swed Dent J (Suppl 11), 1982.

Ellis EE III, McNamara JA Jr: Components of adult class III malocclusion. J Oral Maxillofac Surg 42:295–305, 1984.

Ellis E III, McNamara JA Jr: Cephalometric reference planes: sella nasion vs. Frankfort horizontal. Int J Adult Orthod Orthognath Surg 3:31, 1988.

El-Mangoury NH, Moussa MM, Mostafa YA, Girgis AS: In-vitro remineralization after ARS. J Clin Orthod 25:75–78, 1991.

El-Mangoury NH, Shaheen SI, Mostafa YA: Landmark identification in computerized posteroanterior cephalometrics. Am J Orthod Dentofacial Orthop 91:57–61, 1987.

Endo K, et al: Effects of titanium nitride coatings on surface and coffosion characteristics of NiTi alloy. Dent Mater J 13:228–239, 1994.

Epker BN, Fish LC: *Dentofacial Deformities: Integrated Orthodontic and Surgical Correction.* Vol II. St. Louis, MO: CV Mosby, 1986.

Erverdi N, et al: A comparison of two different rapid palatal expansion techniques from the point of root resorption. Am J Orthod Dentofacial Orthop 106:47–51, 1994.

Feeney F, Morton J, Burstone CJ: The effect of bracket width on bracket–wire friction (Abstract). J Dent Res 67:1969, 1988.

Fish LC, Epker BN: Prevention of relapse in surgical–orthodontic treatment: Part 2. maxillary superior repositioning. J Clin Orthod 21:33–47, 1987.

Fisher JC: Case report. Am J Orthod Dentofacial Orthop 94:1–9, 1988.

Forsyth DB, Shaw WC, Richmond S, Roberts CT: Digital imaging of cephalometric radiographs: Part 2. image quality. Angle Orthod 66:43–50, 1996.

Fosberg CM: Facial morphology and aging: A longitudinal cephalometric investigation of young adults. Eur J Orthod 7:15–23, 1979.

Frank CA, Nikolai RJ: A comparative study of the frictional resistance between an orthodontic bracket and an arch wire. Am J Orthod 78:593–609, 1980.

Fränkel R: The treatment of class II, division I malocclusion with functional correctors. Am J Orthod 55:265–275, 1969.

Fränkel R: Guidance of eruption without extraction. Transactions of the European Orthodontic Society 303–315, 1971.

Fränkel R: Decrowding during eruption under the screening influence of vestibular shields. Am J Orthod 65:372–406, 1974.

Fränkel R: The applicability of the occipital reference base in cephalometrics. Am J Orthod 77:379–395, 1980.

Fränkel R: A functional approach to treatment of skeletal open bite. Am J Orthod 84:54–68, 1983.

Fricke LL, Rankine CAN: Comparison of electrosurgery with conventional fiberotomies on rotational relapse and gingival tissue in the dog. Am J Orthod Dentofacial Orthop 97: 405–412, 1990.

GAC International: *Bioforce Ionguard Information Pamphlet*. Central Islip, NY: GAC International, 1995.

Gamer LD, Allai WW, Moore BK: A comparison of frictional forces during simulated canine retraction of a continuous edgewise arch wire. Am J Orthod 90:199–203, 1986.

Gavakos K, Witt E: The functional status of orthodontically treated prognathic patients. Eur J Orthod 13:124–128, 1991.

Gazit E, Lieberman MA: Occlusal considerations in orthodontics. J Clin Orthod 11:684–691, 1973.

Gianelli A: *Bidimensional Technique Syllabus*. Boston: Boston University, Department of Orthodontics, 1995.

Gianelly AA, Bednar J, Dietz VS: Japanese NiTi coils used to move molars distally. Am J Orthod Dentofacial Orthop 99:564–566, 1991.

Gianelly AA, Hughes HM, Wohlgemuth P, Gildea G: Condylar position and extraction treatment. Am J Orthod Dentofacial Orthop 93:210–215, 1988.

Glenn G, Sinclair P, Alexander RG: Nonextraction orthodontic therapy: post treatment dental and skeletal stability. Am J Orthod Dentofacial Orthop 92:321–328, 1987.

Goldberg D, Turley PK: Orthodontic space closure of the edentulous maxillary first molar area in adults. Int J Adult Orthod Orthognath Surg 4:255–266, 1989.

Goldin B: Labial root torque: effect on the maxilla and incisor root apex. Am J Orthod Dentofacial Orthop 95:209–210, 1989.

Goldson L, Henriksen CO: Root resorption during Begg treatment: a longitudinal roentgenologic study. Am J Orthod 68:55–66, 1975.

Goldstein RE: *Change Your Smile*. Chicago: Quintessence, 1984.

Goldstein RE, Goldstein CE: Is your case really finished? J Clin Orthod 22:702–713, 1988.

Graber LW: Chin cup therapy for mandibular prognathism. Am J Orthod 72:23–41, 1977.

Graber LW: *Orthodontics: State of the Art, Essence of the Science*. St. Louis, MO: CV Mosby, 1986.

Graber TM: Thumb and finger sucking. Am J Orthod 45:259–264, 1959.

Graber TM, Rakosi T, Petrovic AG: *Dentofacial Orthopedics with Functional Appliances*. St. Louis, MO: CV Mosby, 1985.

Graber TM, Swain BF: *Orthodontics: Current Principles and Techniques*. St. Louis, MO: CV Mosby, 1985.

Greenberg AR, Kusy RP: A survey of specialty coatings for orthodontic wires (Abstract). J Dent Res 58:98, 1979.

Greene CS: Orthodontics, orthodontists and TMD. Summarized by Crouch DL. Pacific Coast Society of Orthodontists Bulletin, Winter, 33–35, 1990.

Greenfield B, Kraus S, Lawrence E, Wolf SL: The influence of cephalostatic ear rods on the positions of the head and neck during postural recordings. Am J Orthod Dentofacial Orthop 95:312–318, 1989.

Grummons DC, van de Coppello Kappeyne MA: A frontal asymmetry analysis. J Clin Orthod 21:448–465, 1987.

Guichet NF, Huffman RW, et al: *Principles of Occlusion: Laboratory and Clinical Teaching Manual.* Sect. VI, part A. 2nd ed. Ohio: H. & R. Press, 1969:7–18.

Guyer EC, Ellis EE III, McNamara JA Jr, Behrents RG: Components of class III malocclusion in juveniles and adolescents. Angle Orthod 56:7–30, 1986.

Guyuron B: Precision rhinoplasty I: the role of life-size photographs and soft-tissue cephalometric analysis. Plast Reconstr Surg 81:489, 1988.

Haas AJ: The treatment of maxillary deficiency by opening the midpalatal suture. Angle Orthod 35:200–217, 1965.

Hamula W, Hamula DW, Brower K: Glass ionomer update. J Clin Orthod 27:420–425, 1993.

Han Sand Quick DC: Nickel–titanium spring properties in a simulated oral environment. Angle Orthod 63:67, 1993.

Harris EF, Baker WC: Loss of root length and bone height before and during treatment in adolescent and adult orthodontic patients. Am J Orthod Dentofacial Orthop 98:463–469, 1990.

Harris EF, Newman SM, Nicholson JA: Nitinol arch wire in a simulated oral environment: changes in mechanical properties. Am J Orthod 93:508–513, 1988.

Harris J: A marking device for equilibration. J Clin Orthod 2:111–113, 1971.

Harry MR, Sims MR: Root resorption in bicuspid intrusion: a scanning electronmicroscopic study. Angle Orthod 52:235–258, 1982.

Haryett RD, et al: Chronic thumb sucking: the psychological effects and relative effectiveness of various methods of treatment. Am J Orthod 53:569–585, 1967.

Heimlich AC: Occlusal equilibration in relation to orthodontic treatment. Dent Clin North Am Nov:807–813, 1960.

Heintze SD, Jost-Brinkmann P-G, Loundos J: Effectiveness of three different types of electric toothbrushes compared with a manual technique in orthodontic patients. Am J Orthod Dentofacial Orthop 110:630–638, 1996.

Hemley S: The incidence of root resorption of vital permanent teeth. J Dent Res 20:133–141, 1941.

Hendrix I, Carels C, Kuijpers-Jagtman AM, Hof MVT: A radiographic study of posterior apical root resorption in orthodontic patients. Am J Orthod Dentofacial Orthop 105:345–349, 1994.

Hilgers JJ: Begin with the end in mind: bioprogressive simplified. J Clin Orthod 9:618–627, 10:716–734, 11:794–804, 12:857–870, 1987.

Hine DL, Owen AH III: The stability of the arch expansion effects of Fränkel appliance therapy. Am J Orthod Dentofacial Orthop 98:437–445, 1990.

Hing NR: The accuracy of computer generated prediction tracings. Int J Oral Maxillofac Surg 18:148–151, 1989.

Hirata RH, Heft NWI, Hernandez B, King GH: Longitudinal study of signs of temporomandibular disorders (TMD) in orthodontically treated and nontreated groups. Am J Orthod Dentofacial Orthop 101:35–40, 1992.

Hollender L, Ronnerman A, Thilander B: Root resorption, marginal bone support and clinical crown length in orthodontically treated patients. Eur J Orthod 2:197–205, 1980.

Howe RP: The bonded Herbst appliance. J Clin Orthod 16:663–667, 1982.

Howe RP: Removable plastic Herbst retainer. J Clin Orthod 21:533–537, 1987.

Howe RP: Lower premolar extraction/removable plastic Herbst treatment for mandibular retrognathia. Am J Orthod Dentofacial Orthop 92:275–285, 1987.

Hurst CL, et al: An evaluation of the shape memory phenomenon of nickel-titanium orthodontic wires. Am J Orthod 98:72–76, 1990.

Ireland AJ, Sherriff M, McDonald F: Effect of bracket and wire composition on frictional forces. Eur J Orthod 13:322–328, 1991.

Irie M, Nakamura S: Orthopedic approach to severe skeletal class III malocclusion. Am J Orthod 67:377–392, 1975.

Jackson CL: Comparison between electric toothbrushing and manual toothbrushing with and without oral irrigation, for oral hygiene of orthodontic patients. Am J Orthod Dentofacial Orthop 99:15–20, 1991.

Jackson GW, Kokich VG, Shapiro PA: Experimental response to anteriorly directed extraoral force in young *Macaca nemestrina*. Am J Orthod 75:319–333, 1979.

Jacobs JD, et al: Control of the transverse dimension with surgery and orthodontics. Am J Orthod Dentofacial Orthop 77:284–306, 1980.

Jacoby B, Viazis AD, Abelson M, Allen EP: Periodontal plastic surgery in orthodontics. J Clin Orthod 27:47–49, 1993.

Janson GRP, Martins DR: Functional analysis and occlusal adjustment in orthodontics: A clinical study. Ortodontia 23:4–15, 1990.

Janson WA: Occlusal adjustment. São Paulo, Brazil: Medisa Editora, 1980:256–282.

Jarvinen S: The relation of the Wits appraisal to the ANB angle: Statistical appraisal. Am J Orthod Dentofacial Orthop 94:432–435, 1988.

Johnson D, Smith R: Smile esthetics after orthodontic treatment with and without extraction of four first premolars. Am J Orthod Dentofacial Orthop 108:162–167, 1995.

Johnson E, Lee RS: Relative stiffness of orthodontic wires. J Clin Orthod 23:353–363, 1989.

Johnston LE: *New Vistas in Orthodontics.* Philadelphia: Lea & Febiger, 1985.

Kambara T: Dentofacial changes produced by extra-oral forward force in the *Macaca irus.* Am J Orthod 71:249–277, 1977.

Kapila S, et al: Evaluation of friction between edgewise stainless steel brackets and orthodontic wires of four alloys. Am J Orthod 98:117–126, 1990.

Kapila S, Sachdeva R: Mechanical properties and clinical application of orthodontic wires. Am J Orthod Dentofacial Orthop 96:100, 1989.

Kaplan R: Mandibular third molars and postretention crowding. Am J Orthod 66:411–430, 1974.

Kaplan RG: Induced condylar growth in a patient with hemifacial microsomia. Angle Orthod 59:85–90, 1990.

Katona TR, Moore BK: The effects of load misalignment on tensile load testing of direct bonded orthodontic brackets: a finite element model. Am J Orthod 105:543–551, 1994.

Kennedy DB, Joondeph DR, Osterberg SK, Little RM: The effect of extraction and orthodontic treatment on dentoalveolar support. Am J Orthod 84:183–190, 1983.

Kerosuo H, et al: Nickel allergy in adolescents in relation to orthodontic treatment and piercing of ears. Am J Orthod Dentofacial Orthop 109:148–154, 1996.

Kerr WJS, O'Donnell JM: Panel perception of facial attractiveness. Br J Orthod 17:299–304, 1990.

Ketcham AH: A preliminary report of an investigation of apical root resorption of vital permanent teeth. Int J Orthod 13:97–127, 1927.

Ketcham AH: A progress report of an investigation of apical root resorption of vital permanent teeth. Int J Orthod 15:310–328, 1929.

Khier SE, Brantley WA, Foumelle RA: Bending properties of superelastic and nonsuperelastic nickel-titanium orthodontic wires. Am J Orthod 99:310–318, 1991.

Kinsella P: Some aspects of root resorption in orthodontics. N Z Orthod J: 21–25, 1971.

Kokich VG, Shapiro PA: Lower incisor extraction in orthodontic treatment. Angle Orthod 54:139–154, 1984.

Konstantiantos KA, O'Reilly MT, Close J: The validity of the prediction of soft tissue profile changes after LeFort I osteotomy using the dentofacial planner (computer software). Am J Orthod Dentofacial Orthop 105:241–249, 1994.

Krebs A: Expansion of the midpalatal suture studied by means of metallic implants. Transactions of the European Orthodontic Society 34:163–171, 1958.

Krebs AA: Expansion of midpalatal suture studied by means of metallic implants. Acta Odontol Scand 17:491–501, 1959.

Krebs AA: Rapid expansion of midpalatal suture by fixed appliance: An implant study over a 7 year period. Transactions of the European Orthodontist Society 40:141–142, 1964.

Kundinger KK, Austin BP, Christensen LV, Donegan SJ, Ferguson DJ: An evaluation of TMJ and jaw muscles after orthodontic treatment involving premolar extractions. Am J Orthod Dentofacial Orthop 100:110–115, 1991.

Kurol J, Owman-Moll P, Lundgren D: Time-related root resorption after application of a controlled continuous orthodontic force. Am J Orthod Dentofacial Orthop 110:303–310, 1996.

Kusy RP: Comparison of nickel-titanium and beta-titanium wire sizes to conventional orthodontic archwire materials. Am J Orthod 79:625–629, 1981.

Kusy RP, et al: Surface roughness of orthodontic archwires via laser spectroscopy. Angle Orthod 58:33–45, 1988.

Kusy RP, Greenberg AR: Effects of composition and cross section on the elastic properties of orthodontic archwires. Angle Orthod 51:325–341, 1981.

Kusy RP, Greenberg AR: Comparison of the elastic properties of nickel-titanium and beta-titanium archwires. Am J Orthod 82:199–205, 1982.

Kusy RP, Tobin EJ, Whitley JQ, Sioshansi P: Frictional coefficents of ion-implanted aluminum against ion-implanted beta-titanium in the low load, low velocity, single pass regime. Dental Materials 167–172, 1992.

Kusy RP, Whitley JQ: Effects of sliding velocity on the coefficient of friction in a model orthodontic system. J Dent Mater 5:235–240, 1989.

Kusy RP, Whitley JQ: Coefficients of friction for archwires in stainless steel and polycrystalline alumina bracket slots: 1. the dry state. Am J Orthod 98:300–312, 1990.

Kusy RP, Whitley JQ: Effects of surface roughness on the coefficients of friction in model orthodontic systems. J Biomech 23:913–925, 1993.

Kusy RP, Whitley JQ, Prewitt MJ: Comparison of the frictional coefficents for selected archwire-bracket slot combinations in the dry and wet states. Angle Orthod 61:293–302, 1991.

Kuyl M, et al: The integumental profile: a reflection of the underlying skeletal configuration? Am J Orthod Dentofacial Orthop 106:597–604, 1994.

Kvam E: Scanning electron microscopy of tissue changes on the pressure surface of human premolars following tooth movement. Scand J Dent Res 80:368–375, 1972.

LaFerla MR: *Ion-Implantation: Effect on Frictional Resistance to Movement.* Master's thesis presented to the Faculty of the Graduate School of the University of Southern California, Los Angeles, 1996.

Langer B, Langer L: Subepithelial connective tissue graft technique for root coverage. J Periodontal 56:715, 1985.

Langford NM Jr: The Herbst appliance. J Clin Orthod 15:558–561, 1981.

Langford NM Jr.: Updating fabrication of the Herbst appliance. J Clin Orthod 16:173–174, 1982.

Lapedes DN, et al: *Dictionary of Physics and Mathematics.* 2nd ed. New York: McGraw-Hill, 1978.

Lazarus AH: Precision grinding. J Clin Orthod 6:332–334, 1971.

Levander E, Malmgren O: Evaluation of the risk of root resorption during orthodontic treatment: a study of upper incisors. Eur J Orthod 10:30–38, 1988.

Lines PA, Lines RR, Lines C: Profile metrics and facial esthetics. Am J Orthod 73:648, 1978.

Linge BO, Linge L: Apical root resorption in upper anterior teeth. Eur J Orthod 5:173–183, 1983.

Litt RA, Nielsen IL: Class II, division 2 malocclusion: to extract or not extract? Angle Orthod 54:123–138, 1984.

Little R: Stability and relapse of dental arch alignment. Br J Orthod 17:235–241, 1990.

Little R, Riedel R: Postretention evaluation of stability and relapse: mandibular arches with generalized spacing. Am J Orthod Dentofacial Orthop 95:37–41, 1989.

Little R, Riedel R, Artun J: An evaluation of changes in mandibular anterior alignment from 10 to 20 years postretention. Am J Orthod Dentofacial Orthop 93:423–428, 1988.

Little R, Riedel R, Engst D: Serial extraction of first bicuspids: postretention evaluation of stability and relapse. Angle Orthod 60:255–326, 1991.

Little R, Riedel R, Stein A: Mandibular arch length increase during the mixed dentition: postretention evaluation of stability and relapse. Am J Orthod Dentofacial Orthop 97: 393–404, 1990.

Little R, Waller T, Riedel R: Stability and relapse of mandibular anterior alignment: first bicuspid extraction cases treated by traditional edgewise orthodontic. Am J Orthod 80:349–365, 1981.

Little RM: Orthodontic stability and relapse. Summary by Bergh HC. Pacific Coast Society of Orthodontists Bulletin, 35–38, 1991.

Liveratos F, Johnston L: A comparison of one-stage and two-stage nonextraction alternatives in matched class-II samples. Am J Orthod Dentofacial Orthop 108:118–131, 1995.

Lopez I, Goldberg J, Burstone CJ: Bending characteristics of nitinol wire. Am J Orthod 75:569–575, 1979.

Luecke PE III, Johnston LE Jr: The effect of maxillary first premolar extraction and incisor retraction on mandibular position: testing the central dogma of "functional orthodontics." Am J Orthod Dentofacial Orthop 101:4–12, 1992.

Lundström A: Guest editorial: intercranial reference lines versus the true horizontal as a basis for cephalometric analysis. Eur J Orthod 13:167–168, 1991.

Lundström A, Fosberg CM, Westergren H, Lundström F: A comparison between estimated and registered NHP. Eur J Orthod 13:59–64, 1991.

Lundström A, Lundström F: The Frankfort horizontal as a basis for cephalometric analysis. Am J Orthod Dentofacial Orthop 107:537–540, 1995.

Lundström F, Lundström A: Clinical evaluation of maxillary and mandibular prognathism. Eur J Orthod 11:408–413, 1989.

Lupi J, et al: Prevalence and severity of apocol root resorption and alveolar bone loss in orthodontically treated adults. Am J Orthod Dentofacial Orthop 109:28–37, 1996.

Luyk NP, Whitfield PH, Ward-Booth RP, Williams ED: The reproducibility of the natural head position in lateral cephalometric radiographs. Br J Oral Maxillofac Surg 24:357–366, 1986.

MacDonald S, Bums D: *Physics for the Life and Health Sciences.* New York: Addison-Wesley, 1975.

Maessa R, et al: Long-term stability of rapid palatal expander treatment and eclusive mechanotherapy. Am J Orthod Dentofacial Orthop 108:478–488, 1995.

Maijer R, Smith DC: A comparison between zinc phosphate and glass ionomer cement in orthodontics. Am J Orthod 93:273–279, 1988.

Mamandras AH, Allen LP: Mandibular response to orthodontic treatment with the Bionator appliance. Am J Orthod Dentofacial Orthop 97:113–120, 1990.

Manhartsberger C, Seidenbusch W: Force delivery of N. J. coil springs. Am J Orthod Dentofacial Orthop 109:8–21, 1996.

Marry MR, Sims MR: Root resorption in bicuspid intrusion: a scanning electron microscope study. Angle Orthod 52:235–258, 1982.

Marshall JA: A comparison of resorption of roots of deciduous teeth with the absorption of roots of the permanent teeth occurring as a result of infection. Int J Orthod 15:417, 1929.

Marshall JS, Pounder ER, Stewart RW: *Physics.* 2nd ed. New York: The MacMillan Co, 1967.

Massler M, Malone AJ: Root resorption in human permanent teeth. Am J Orthod 40: 619–633, 1954.

Massler M, Perreault JG: Root resorption in the permanent teeth of young adults. J Dent Child 21:158–164, 1954.

McFadden WM, Engström C, Engström H, Anholm JM: A study of the relationship between incisor intrusion and root shortening. Am J Orthod Dentofacial Orthop 96:390–396, 1989.

McHorris WH: Occlusion: with particular emphasis on the functional and parafunctional role of anterior teeth. J Clin Orthod 13:606–620, 1979.

McIver LN: Five steps to better occlusion in class II treatment. Am J Orthod 48:175–190, 1962.

McLaughlin RP, Bennet TC: The transition from standard edgewise to preadjusted appliance systems. J Clin Orthod 23:142–153, 1989.

McLaughlin RP, Bennett JC: Anchorage control during leveling and aligning with a preadjusted appliance system. J Clin Orthod 25:687–696, 1991.

McNamara JA Jr: *Neuromuscular and Skeletal Adaptations to Altered Orofacial Function*. Ann Arbor, MI: Monograph 1, Craniofacial Growth Series, Center for Human Growth and Development, University of Michigan, 1972.

McNamara JA Jr: Functional determinants of craniofacial size and shape. Eur J Orthod 2:131–159, 1980.

McNamara JA Jr: An orthopedic approach to the treatment of class III malocclusion in young patients. J Clin Orthod 21:598–608, 1987.

McNamara JA Jr, Brudon WL: *Orthodontic and Orthopedic Treatment in the Mixed Dentition*. Ann Arbor, MI: Needham Press, 1993.

McNamara JA Jr, Carlson DS: Quantitative analysis of temporomandibular joint adaptations to protrusive function. Am J Orthod 76:593–611, 1979.

McNamara JA Jr, Connelly T, McBride MC: *Histological Studies of Temporomandibular Joint Adaptations: Determinants of Mandibular Form and Growth*. Ann Arbor, MI: Monograph 4, Craniofacial Growth Series, Center for Human Growth and Development, University of Michigan, 1975.

McNamara JA Jr, Ellis E III: Cephalometric analysis of untreated adults with ideal facial and occlusal relationships. Int J Adult Orthod Orthognath Surg 3:221, 1988.

McNeill RW, Joondeph DR: Congenitally absent maxillary lateral incisors: treatment planning considerations. Angle Orthod 43:24–29, 1973.

McReynolds DC, Little RM: Mandibular second bicuspid extraction: postretention evaluation of stability and relapse. Angle Orthod 61:133–144, 1991.

Melsen B: The cranial base: the postnatal development of the cranial base studied histologically on human autopsy material. Acta Odontol Scand Suppl 32:62, 1974.

Melsen, B: *Current Controversies in Orthodontics*. Chicago: Quintessence Publishing, 1991.

Melsen B, Bjerrejaard J, Bundgaard M: The effect of treatment with functional appliance on a pathologic growth pattern of the condyle. Am J Orthod 90:503, 1986.

Meng HP, Goorhuls J, Kapila S, Narida RS: Growth changes in the nasal profile from 7 to 18 years of age. Am J Orthod 94:917–926, 1988.

Mermigos J, Full CA, Andreasen G: Protraction of the maxillofacial complex. Am J Orthod Dentofacial Orthop 98:47–55, 1990.

Michiels LYF, Tourne LPM: Nasion true vertical: a proposed method for testing the clinical validity of cephalometric measurements applied to a new cephalometric reference line. Int J Adult Orthod Orthognath Surg 5:43–52, 1990.

Miller EL, Bodden WR, Jamison HC: A study of the relationship of the dental midline to the facial median line. J Prosthet Dent 41:657, 1979.

Miller F: *College Physics*. 4th ed. New York: Harcourt, Brace, Jovanovich, 1977.

Miller PD Jr: Root coverage using a free soft tissue autograft following citric acid application: I. technique. Int J Periodontal Rest Dent 2:65, 1982.

Mirabella A, Artun J: Risk factors for apical root resorption of maxillary anterior teeth in adult orthodontic patients. Am J Orthod Dentofacial Orthop 108:48–55, 1995.

Mitani H: Occlusal and craniofacial growth changes during puberty. Am J Orthod 72:76–84, 1977.

Mitani H: Prepubertal growth of mandibular prognathism. Am J Orthod 80:546–553, 1981.

Mitani H, Sakamoto T: Chin cup force to a growing mandible. Angle Orthod 54:93–122, 1984.

Miura F: Reflections on my involvement in orthodontic research. Am J Orthod Dentofacial Orthop 104:531, 1993.

Miura F, et al: The super-elastic property of the Japanese NiTi alloy wire for use in orthodontics. Am J Orthod 90:1–10, 1986.

Miura F, Masakuri M, Yasuo O: New application of the superelastic NiTi rectangular wire. J Clin Orthod 24:544–548, 1990.

Miura F, Mogi M, Ohura Y, Karibe M: The super-elastic Japanese NiTi alloy wire for use in orthodontics. Am J Orthod Dentofacial Orthop 94:89–96, 1988.

Mohl ND, Zarb GA, Carlsson GE, Rugh JD: *A Textbook of Occlusion*. Chicago: Quintessence Publishing, 1988.

Moon HB: *Evaluation of Frictional Resistance Between Orthodontic Brackets and Arch Wires in Relation to the Coefficient of Friction and the Modulus of Elasticisty*. Master's Thesis, University of Southern California, Los Angeles, 1992.

Moon HB, Zemik JH: Modeling of resistance to sliding between orthodontic brackets (Abstract). J Dent Res 71:89, 1992.

Moorrees CFA, Kean MR: Natural head position, a basic consideration in the interpretation of cephalometric radiographs. Am J Phys Anthropol 16:213–223, 1988.

Morgan J: *Introduction to University Physics*. Vol 1. 2nd ed. Allyn and Bacon, 1969.

Moskowitz ME, Nayyar A: Determinants of dental esthetics: a rationale for smile analysis and treatment. Compendium 16:1164–1186, 1995.

Moyers RE: Pasos clinicos propuestos para obviar la recidiva ortodonica. Ortodonica 34: 238–253, 1970.

Nanda R: Protraction of maxilla in rhesus monkeys by controlled extraoral forces. Am J Orthod 74:121–131, 1978.

Nanda R: Biomechanical and clinical considerations of a modified protraction headgear. Am J Orthod 78:125–138, 1980.

Newman WG: Possible etiologic factors in external root resorption. Am J Orthod 67: 522–539, 1975.

Nfiura F, Mogi M, Ohura Y, Hamanaka H: The superelastic property of the Japanese NiTi alloy wire for use in orthodontics. Am J Orthod 90:1–10, 1986.

Ngan P, et al: Soft tissue and dentoskeletal profile changes associated with maxillary expansion and protraction headgear treatment. Am J Orthod Dentofacial Orthop 109:38–49, 1996.

Ngan P, Wilson S, Shanfeld J, Amini H: The effect of ibuprofen on the level of discomfort in patients undergoing orthodontic treatment. Am J Orthod Dentofacial Orthop 106:88, 1994.

Nicholls J: Frictional forces in fixed orthodontic appliances. Dent Pract Dent Rec 18:362–366, 1968.

Nordquist GG, McNeill RW: Orthodontic vs. restorative treatment of the congenitally absent lateral incisor: long term periodontal and occlusal evaluation. J Periodontol 46:139–143, 1975.

Oakes C, Hatcher JE: Determining physiologic archforms. J Clin Orthod 25:79–80, 1991.

Ogaard B, Rolla G, Arends J: Orthodontic appliances and enamel demineralization. Am J Orthod Dentofacial Orthop 94:68–73, 1988.

Okeson JP: *Management of Temporomandibular Disorders and Occlusion*. 2nd ed. St. Louis, MO: Mosby, 1989.

Oktay, H: A comparison of ANB, WITS, AF-BF, and APDI measurements. Am J Orthod Dentofacial Orthop 99:122–128, 1991.

Omana HM, Moore RN, Bagby MD: Frictional properties of metal and ceramic brackets. J Clin Orthod 26:342–425, 1992.

Oppenheim A: Biologic orthodontic therapy and reality: part III. Angle Orthod 6:69–116, 1936.

Orchin JD: Permanent lingual bonded retainer. J Clin Orthod 24:229–231, 1991.

O'Reilly M, et al: Class II elastics and extractions and temporomandibular disorders: a longitudinal prospective study. Am J Orthod Dentofacial Orthop 103:459–463, 1993.

O'Reilly MM, Featherstone JDB: Demineralization and remineralization around orthodontic appliances: an in vitro study. Am J Orthod Dentofacial Orthop 92:33–40, 1987.

Orthodontic Dialogue: *Teamwork Enhances Patient Esthetics*. Vol. 2, Number 2, Spring, 1990.

Page R: Frontiers in periodontics. Summary by Nichols O. Pacific Coast Society of Orthodontists Bulletin, Spring, 39–41, 1991.

Pancherz H: Treatment of class II malocclusions by jumping the bite with the Herbst appliance: a cephalometric investigation. Am J Orthod 76:423–441, 1979.

Pancherz H: A cephalometric long-term investigation on the nature of class II relapse after Herbst appliance treatment. Am J Orthod Dentofacial Orthop 100:220–233, 1991.

Pancherz H, Anehus-Pancherz J: Muscle activity in class II, division 1 malocclusions treated by jumping the bite with the Herbst appliance: an electromyographic study. Am J Orthod 78:321–329, 1980.

Pancherz H, Anehus-Pancherz J: The effect of continuous bite jumping with the Herbst appliance on the masticatory system: a functional analysis of treated class II malocclusions. Eur J Orthod 4:37–44, 1982.

Pancherz H, Fackel V: The skeletofacial growth pattern pre- and post-dentofacial orthopaedics: a long-term study of class II malocclusions treated with the Herbst appliance. Eur J Orthod 12:209–218, 1990.

Parker WS: Centric relation and centric occlusion: an orthodontic responsibility. Am J Orthod Dentofacial Orthop 74:481–500, 1978.

Pearson LE: Vertical control in fully-banded orthodontic treatment. Angle Orthod 205R–224, 1986.

Perkins R, Staley R: Change in lip vermilion height during orthodontic treatment. Am J Orthod Dentofacial Orthop 103:147–154, 1993.

Peterson L, et al: A comparison of friction resistance for nitinol and stainless steel wire in edgewise brackets. Quin Int 13:563–571, 1982.

Phillips C, Hill BJ, Cannac C: The influence of video imaging on patients' perceptions and expectations. Angle Orthod 65:263–270, 1995.

Phillips JR: Apical root resorption under orthodontic therapy. Angle Orthod 25:1–22, 1955.

Polson AM, Subtenly JD, Heitner SW, Polson AP, Sommers EW, Iker HP, Reed BE: Long-term periodontal status after orthodontic treatment. Am J Orthod Dentofacial Orthop 93:51–58, 1988.

Popovich F, Thompson GW: Thumb and finger sucking: its relation to malocclusion. Am J Orthod 63:148–155, 1973.

Popp TW, et al: Nonsurgical treatment for a class III dental relationship: a case report. Am J Orthod 103:203–211, 1993.

Posen TM: Longitudinal study of the growth of the nose. Am J Orthod 53:746–756, 1967.

Pound E: *Personalized Denture Procedures: Dentist's Manual*. Anaheim, CA: Denar, 1973.

Pratten DH, et al: Frictional resistance of ceramic and stainless steel orthodontic brackets. Am J Orthod 98:398–403, 1990.

Proffit WR: *Contemporary Orthodontics*. St. Louis, MO: CV Mosby, 1984.

Proffit WR: *Contemporary Orthodontics*. St. Louis, MO: CV Mosby, 1986.

Proffit, WR: *Contemporary Orthodontics*. 2nd ed. St. Louis, MO: Mosby, 1992.

Proffit WR: *Contemporary Orthodontics*. 2nd ed. St. Louis, MO: Mosby-Year Book, 1993.

Proffit WR, White RP: *Surgical–Orthodontic Treatment.* St. Louis, MO: Mosby-Year Book, 1991.

Prososki RR, Bagby, MD, Erickson LC: Static frictional force and surface roughness of nickel-titanium arch wires. Am J Orthod 100:341–348, 1991.

Radlanski RJ, Jager A, Schwestka R, Bertzbach F: Plaque accumulation caused by interdental stripping. Am J Orthod 94:416–420, 1988.

Randow K, et al: The effect of an occlusal interference on the masticatory system. Odontol Rev 27:245–256, 1976.

Reitan K: Effects of force magnitude and directions of tooth movement on different alveolar bone types. Angle Orthod 34:244–255, 1964.

Reitan K: Initial tissue behavior during apical root resorption. Angle Orthod 44:68–82, 1974.

Reitan K: Biomechanical principles and reactions: In: Graber TM, Swain BF, eds. *Orthodontics: Current Principles and Techniques.* St. Louis, MO: CV Mosby, 1985: 101–192.

Rendell JK, Norton LA, Gay T: Orthodontic treatment and temporomandibular joint disorders. Am J Orthod Dentofacial Orthop 101:84–87, 1992.

Ricketts RM: Planning treatment on the basis of the facial pattern and an estimate of its growth. Angle Orthod 43:105–119, 1957.

Ricketts RM: Perspectives in clinical application of cephalometrics. Angle Orthod 29:93–104, 1959.

Ricketts RM: The influence of orthodontic treatment on facial growth and development. Angle Orthod 30:103–133, 1960.

Ricketts RM: A foundation of cephalometric communication. Am J Orthod 46:330–357, 1960.

Ricketts RM: Cephalometric analysis and synthesis. Am J Orthod 31:141–156, 1961.

Ricketts RM: The value of cephalometrics and computerized technology. Angle Orthod 42:179–199, 1972.

Ricketts RM: Perspectives in clinical application of cephalometrics. Angle Orthod 51: 115–150, 1981.

Riley JL, Garrett SG, Moon PC: Frictional forces of ligated plastic and metal edgewise brackets. J Dent Res 58:A21, 1979.

Roberts WW, et al: A segmental approach to mandibular molar uprighting. Am J Orthod Dentofacial Orthop 81:177–184, 1982.

Roche AF, Lewis, AB: Late growth changes in the cranial base. In: Bosma JF, ed. *Development of the Basicranium.* Bethesda, MD: DHEW Publications, 1976: 221–239.

Rose CM: *Evaluation of Resistance Forces Between Ceramic Brackets and Orthodontic Wire.* Master's Thesis, University of Southern California, Los Angeles, 1995.

Rose CM, Zemik JH: Reduced resistance to sliding in ceramic brackets. J Clin Orthod 30:78–84, 1996.

Rosenberg HN: An evaluation of the incidence and amount of apical root resorption and dilaceration occurring in orthodontically treated teeth, having incompletely formed roots at the beginning of Begg treatment. Am J Orthod 61:524–525, 1972.

Roth PM, et al: Congenitally missing lateral incisor treatment. J Clin Orthod 4:258–262, 1985.

Roth RH: Temporomandibular pain–dysfunction and occlusal relationships. Angle Orthod 43:136–153, 1973.

Roth RH: Functional occlusion for the orthodontist: Part 1. J Clin Orthod 15:32–51, 1981.

Roth RH: Functional occlusion for the orthodontist: Part 3. J Clin Orthod 3:174–198, 1981.

Roth RH: Treatment mechanics for the straight wire appliance. In: Graber TM, Swain BF, eds. *Orthodontics: Current Principles and Techniques.* St. Louis, MO: CV Mosby, 1985: 665–716.

Roth RH, Rolfs DA: Functional occlusion for the orthodontist: Part II. J Clin Orthod 15:100–123, 1981.

Rudee DA: Proportional profile changes concurrent with orthodontic therapy. Am J Orthod 50:421, 1964.

Rudolph CE: A comparative study in root resorption in permanent teeth. J Am Dent Assoc 23:822–826, 1936.

Rudolph CE: An evaluation of root resorption occurring during orthodontic treatment. J Dent Res 19:367–371, 1940.

Rushton R, Cohen AM, Linney AD: The relationship and reproducibility of angle ANB and the Wits appraisal. Br J Orthod 18:225–231, 1991.

Rutter RR, Witt E: Correction of class II, division 2 malocclusions through the use of the Bionator appliance. Am J Orthod Dentofacial Orthop 97:106–112, 1990.

Sadowsky C, et al: Long-term stability after orthodontic treatment: nonextraction with prolonged retention. Am J Orthod Dentofacial Orthop 106:243–249, 1994.

Sadowsky C, Poison AM: Temporomandibular disorders and functional occlusion after orthodontic treatment: Results of two long-term studies. Am J Orthod Dentofacial Orthop 86: 386–390, 1984.

Sadowsky C, Theisen TA, Sakols EI: Orthodontic treatment and TMJ sounds: A longitudinal study. Am J Orthod Dentofacial Orthop 99:441–447, 1991.

Sakamoto T: Effective timing for the application of orthopedic force in the skeletal class III malocclusion. Am J Orthod 80:411–416, 1981.

Salzmann JA: Pollock Tribute: Orthodontics in practice and perspective. Am J Orthod Dentofacial Orthop 55:10–19, 1969.

Samas KV, Solow B: Early adult changes in the skeletal and soft tissue profile. Eur J Orthod 2:1–12, 1980.

Sandler J, DiBiase, D: The inclined biteplane: a useful tool. Am Orthod Dentofacial Orthop 110:339–350, 1996.

Sarver DM: Video imaging: a computer facilitated approach to communication and planning in orthognathic surgery. Br J Orthod 20:187–191, 1993.

Sarver DM: Video cephalometric diagnosis (VCD): a new concept in treatment planning. Am J Orthod Dentofacial Orthop 110:128–136, 1996.

Sarver DM, Johnston MW: Orthognathic surgery and esthetics: planning treatment to achieve functional and esthetic goals. Br J Orthod 20:93–100, 1993.

Sarver DM, Johnston MW, Matukas VJ: Video imaging for planning and counseling in orthognathic surgery. J Oral Maxillofac Surg 46:939–945, 1988.

Schluger S: Periodontal aspects of orthodontic treatment. J Clin Orthod 3:111–117, 1968.

Schuberth G, et al: Case report: mandibular advancement and reduction genioplasty. Am J Orthod Dentofacial Orthop 98:481–487, 1990.

Schwartz AM: Tissue changes incidental to tooth movement. Int J Orthod 18:331–352, 1932.

Schwartz ML, Phillips RW, Clark HE: Long term fluoride release from glass ionomer cements. J Dent Res 63:158–160, 1984.

Sears F, Zemansky M, Young H: *University Physics.* 6th ed. New York: Addison-Wesley, 1982.

Seely DM: Treatment of crowded class II malocclusion: case report. Am J Orthod Dentofacial Orthop 104:298–303, 1993.

Selwyn-Bamett BJ: Rationale of treatment for class II, division 2 malocclusion. Br J Orthod 18:173–181, 1991.

Senty EL: The maxillary cuspid and missing lateral incisors: Esthetics and occlusion. Angle Orthod 46:365–371, 1976.

Shafer WG, Hine MK, Levi BM: *A Textbook of Oral Pathology.* 4th ed. Philadelphia: WB Saunders, 1983:328–332.

Shannon IL: Prevention of decalcification in orthodontic patients. J Clin Orthod 15:695–705, 1981.

Sharpe W, Reed B, Subtelny JD, Polson A: Orthodontic relapse, apical root resorption, and crestal alveolar bone levels. Am J Orthod Dentofacial Orthop 91:252–258, 1987.

Shelton C, et al: Decrease treatment time due to changes in technique and practice philosophy. Am J Orthod Dentofacial Orthop 106:654–657, 1994.

Sheridan JJ: Air-rotor stripping. J Clin Orthod 19:43–59, 1985.

Sheridan JJ: Air-rotor stripping update. J Clin Orthod 21:781–788, 1987.

Sheridan JJ, et al: Finishing and retention. J Clin Orthod 9:551–564, 1992.

Sheridan J, LeDoux W, McMinn R: Essix Retainers: Fabrication and Supervision for Permanent Retention. J Clin Orthop 27:37–45, 1993.

Sheridan J, LeDoux W, McMinn R: Essix technology for the fabrication of temporary anterior bridges. J Clin Orthop 28: 482–486, 1994.

Sherman SL, Woods M, Nanda RS: The longitudinal effects of growth on the Wits appraisal. Am J Orthod Dentofacial Orthop 93:429–436, 1988.

Showfety KJ, Vig PS, Matteson SA: A simple method for taking natural-head-position cephalograms. Am J Orthod 83:495–500, 1983.

Siersbaek-Nielsen S, Solow B: Intra- and interexaminer variability in head posture recorded by dental auxiliaries. Am J Orthod 82:50–57, 1982.

Sinclair P, Little R: Maturation of untreated normal occlusions. Am J Orthod 83:114–123, 1983.

Sinclair PM, Kilpelainen P, Phillips C, White RP, Rogers L, Sarver DM: The accuracy of video imaging in orthognathic surgery. Am J Orthod Dentofacial Orthop 107:177–185, 1995.

Sjolien T, Zachrisson BU: Periodontal bone support and tooth length in orthodontically treated and untreated persons. Am J Orthod 64:28–37, 1973.

Smith V, et al: Rigid internal fixation and the effects on the temporomandibular joint and masticatory system: a prospective study. Am J Orthod Dentofacial Orthop 102:491–500, 1992.

Solow B, Siersbaek-Nielsen S, Greeve E: Airway adequacy, head posture, and craniofacial morphology: Part 1. Am J Orthod 86:495–500, 1983.

Solow B, Siersbaek-Nielsen S, Greeve E: Airway adequacy, head posture, and craniofacial morphology: Part 2. Am J Orthod 86:214–223, 1984.

Solow B, Tallgren A: Natural head position in standing subjects. Acta Odontol Scand 29:591–607, 1971.

Solow B, Tallgren A: Head posture and craniofacial morphology. Am J Phys Anthropol 44:417–436, 1976.

Sonis AL: Comparison of NiTi coil springs vs. elastics in canine retraction. J Clin Orthod 28:293, 1994.

Spillers JD: An In Vitro Evaluation of the Force Delivered by Three Japanese Nickel-Titanium Alloy Wires Using the Three-Point Bend Test. Master's Thesis. Kansas City, MO: University of Missouri, Kansas City, 1993.

Spring HB: Comparison of the five analytic reference lines of the horizontal lip position: their consistency and sensitivity. Am J Orthod Dentofacial Orthop 104:355–360, 1993.

Staggers J: Vertical changes following first premolar extractions. Am J Orthod Dentofacial Orthop 105:19–24, 1994.

Stannard JG, Gau JM, Hanna MA: Comparative friction of orthodontic wires under dry and wet conditions. Am J Orthod 89:485–491, 1986.

Steffen JM, Haltom FT: The five cent tooth positioner. J Clin Orthod 21:525–529, 1987.

Steiner CC: Cephalometrics for you and me. Am J Orthod Dentofacial Orthop 39:729–755, 1953.

Stella JP, Epker BN: Systematic aesthetic evaluation of the nose for cosmetic surgery. Oral Maxillofac Surg Clin North Am 2:273, 1990.

Stenvik A, Mjör I: Pulp and dentine reactions to experimental tooth intrusion: a histologic study of the initial changes. Am J Orthod 57:370–385, 1970.

Stepovich ML: A clinical study on closing edentulous spaces in the mandible. Angle Orthod 49:227–233, 1979.

Stockli PW, Wiflert HG: Tissue reactions in the temporomandibular joint resulting from anterior displacement of the mandible in the monkey. Am J Orthod 60:142–155, 1971.

Subtenly JD: A longitudinal study of soft tissue facial structures and their profile characteristics defined in relation to underlying skeletal structures. Am J Orthod 45:481–507, 1959.

Subtenly JD: The soft tissue profile, growth and treatment changes. Angle Orthod 31: 105–122, 1961.

Sugawara J, Asano T, Endo N, Mitani H: Long-term effects of chin cup therapy on skeletal profile in mandibular prognathism. Am J Orthod Dentofacial Orthop 98:127–133, 1990.

Swain BF: Straight wire design strategies: five-year evaluation of the Roth modification of the Andrews straight wire appliance. In: Graber LW, ed. *Orthodontics: State of the Art, Essence of the Science*. St. Louis, MO: CV Mosby, 1986:279–298.

Swartz ML: Orthodontic archwires: a contemporary view. In: *Contemporary Edgewise Syllabus*.

Syliangco SM, Sameshima GTI, Kaminishi RM, Sinclair PM: The accuracy of video imaging in the prediction of mandibular advancement surgery. Angle Orthod 1996 (in press).

Tager BN: Endocrine problems in orthodontics. Am J Orthod 37:867–875, 1951.

Taithongchai R, et al: Facial and dentoalveolar structure and the prediction of apical root shortening. Am J Orthod Dentofacial Orthop 110:296–302, 1996.

Tedesco LA, et al: A dental–facial attractiveness scale. Am J Orthod 83:38–43, 1983.

Teuscher U: A growth-related concept for skeletal class II treatment. Am J Orthod 74:258–275, 1978.

Teuscher U: An appraisal of growth and reaction to extraoral anchorage. Am J Orthod 89:113–121, 1986.

Teuscher U, Stockli P: Combined activator, headgear orthopedics. In: *Orthodontics: Current Principles and Techniques*. St. Louis, MO: CV Mosby, 1985:405–480.

Thilander BL: Complications of orthodontic treatment. Orthop Pediatr 2(5):28–37, 1992.

Thompson JR: Function: the neglected phase of orthodontics. Angle Orthod 26:129–143, 1956.

Thompson JR: Abnormal function of the stomatognathic system and its orthodontic implications. Am J Orthod 48:758–765, 1962.

Thompson JR: Abnormal function of the temporomandibular joints and musculature: Part 3. Am J Orthod Dentofacial Orthop 105:224–240, 1994.

Tidy DC: Frictional forces in fixed appliances. Am J Orthod 96:249–254, 1989.

Tonner RIM, Waters NE: The characteristics of super-elastic NiTi wires in threepoint bending: Part I. the effect of temperature. Eur J Orthod 16:409–419, 1994.

Tonner RIM, Waters NE: The characteristics of super-elastic NiTi wires in threepoint bending: Part II. intra-batch variation. Eur J Orthad 16:421–425, 1994.

Trig T, et al: Effect of head posture on cephalometric sagittal angular measures. Am J Orthod Dentofacial Orthop 104:337–341, 1993.

Trotter J: *An Analysis and Comparison of the Resistance to Movement of an Archwire Through a Bracket with a Stainless Steel, Teflon-Coated, or Elastic Ligature*. Master's Thesis. University of Southern California, Los Angeles, 1994.

Tselepsis, M, Brockhurst P, West C: The dynamic frictional resistance between orthodontic brackets and arch wires. Am J Orthod Dentofacial Orthop 106:131–138, 1994.

Tselepsi M, et al: The dynamic frictional resistance between orthodontic brackets and arch wires. Am J Orthod Dentofacial Orthop 106:131–138, 1994.

Turley PK: Orthopedic correction of class III malocclusion with palatal expansion and custom protraction headgear. J Clin Orthod 22:314–325, 1988.

Turpin DL: Computers coming on line for diagnosis and treatment planning. (Editorial). Angle Orthod 60:163–164, 1990.

Tuverson DL: Anterior interocclusal relations: Part II. Am J Orthod Dentofacial Orthop 78:371–393, 1980.

Ung N, Koenig T, Shapiro PA, Shapiro G, Trask G: A quantitative assessment of respiratory patterns and their effects on dentofacial development. Am J Orthod Dentofacial Orthop 98:523–532, 1990.

Vadiakas G, Fiazis AD: Anterior crossbite connection in the primary dentition. Am J Orthod Dentofacial Orthop 102:160–162, 1992.

Valant JR, Sinclair PM: Treatment effects of the Herbst appliance. Am J Orthod Dentofacial Orthop 95:138–147, 1989.

Valinoti JR: Mandibular incisor extraction therapy. Am J Orthod Dentofacial Orthop 105:107–116, 1994.

Van Beek H: Combination headgear activator. J Clin Orthod 18:185–189, 1984.

Vardimon AD, Graber TM, Voss LR, Lenke J: Determinants controlling iatrogenic external root resorptions and repair during and after palatal expansion. Angle Orthod 61:113–122, 1991.

Viazis AD: A new measurement of profile esthetics. J Clin Orthod 25:15–20, 1991.

Viazis AD: A cephalometric analysis based on natural head position. J Clin Orthod 25: 172–182, 1991.

Viazis AD: Clinical application of superelastic nickel-titanium wires. J Clin Orthod 25: 370–374, 1991.

Viazis AD: The cranial base triangle. J Clin Orthod 25:565–570, 1991.

Viazis AD: Use of elastics with rectangular NiTi wires. J Clin Orthod 25:697–698, 1991.

Viazis AD: The triple-loop corrector. Am J Orthod Dentofacial Orthop 100:91–92, 1991.

Viazis AD: Anteroposterior assessment of the maxilla and the mandible based on the true horizontal. J Clin Orthod 26:673–680, 1992.

Viazis AD: Orthodontic wires. In: *Atlas of Orthodontics*. Philadelphia: WB Saunders, 1993.

Viazis AD: *Atlas of Orthodontics*. Philadelphia: WB Saunders, 1993.

Viazis AD: Bioefficient therapy. J Clin Orthod 29:552–568, 1995.

Viazis AD: *The Viazis System: Bioefficient Therapy*. Islip, NY: GAC International, 1995.

Vig PS, Showfety KJ, Phillips CP: Experimental manipulation of head posture. Am J Orthod 77:258–268, 1980.

Von der Ahe G: Postretention status of maxillary incisors with root-end resorption. Angle Orthod 43:247–255, 1973.

Wadhwa L, Tewari A: A study of clinical signs and symptoms of temporamandibular dysfunction in subjects with normal occlusion, untreated, and treated malocclusion. Am J Orthod Dentofacial Orthop 103:54–61, 1993.

Wallen T, Bloomquist D: The clinical examination: is it more important than cephalometric analysis in surgical orthodontics? Int J Adult Orthod Orthognath Surg 1:179, 1986.

Watanabe K: Studies on new superelastic NiTi orthodontic wire, Part 1. Japanese Journal of Dental Materials 1:47–57, 1982.

Waters NE, Houston WJB, Stephens CD: The characterization of arch wires for the initial alignment of irregular teeth. Am J Orthod 79:373–389, 1981.

Webster's New World Dictionary. Warner Books, 1984.

Wendell PD, Nanda R, Sakamoto T, Nakamura S: The effects of chin cup therapy on the mandible: A longitudinal study. Am J Orthod 87:265–274, 1985.

Wennström J: Periodontal tissue response to orthodontic movement of teeth with infrabony pockets. Am J Orthod Dentofacial Orthop 103:313–319, 1993.

Wertz RA: Skeletal and dental changes accompanying rapid midpalatal suture opening. Am J Orthod 58:41–66, 1970.

West A, et al: Multiflex versus superelastic: a randomized clinical trial of the tooth alignment ability of initial arch wires. Am J Orthod Dentofacial Orthop 108:464–471, 1995.

White LW: Individualized ideal arches. J Clin Orthod 7A:779–787, 1978.

Wieslander L: Dentofacial orthopedics: headgear-Herbst treatment in the mixed dentition. J Clin Orthod 18:551–564, 1984.

Wieslander L, Lagerstron L: The effect of activator treatment on class II malocclusions. Am J Orthod 75:20–26, 1979.

Wilcoxon DB, Ackerman RJ, Kifloy WJ, Love JW, Sakamura J, Tira DE: The effectiveness of a counterrotational-action power toothbrush on plaque control in orthodontic patients. Am J Orthod Dentofacial Orthop 99:7–14, 1991.

Williams R: Eliminating lower retention. J Clin Orthod 11:342–349, 1985.

Williamson EH: Occlusion: understanding or misunderstanding. Angle Orthod 46:86–93, 1976.

Williamson EH: JCO interviews: Dr. Eugene H. Williamson on occlusion and TMJ dysfunction: Part 1. J Clin Orthod 15:333–350, 1981.

Williamson EH: JCO interviews: Dr. Eugene H. Williamson on occlusion and TMJ dysfunction: Part II. J Clin Orthod 15:393–410, 1981.

Williamson EH, et al: The influence of three types of positioners on mandibular condyle relationships. J Clin Orthod 18:335–341, 1984.

Woodside DG, Metaxas A, Altuna G: The influence of functional appliance therapy on glenoid fossa remodeling. Am J Orthod Dentofacial Orthop 92:181–189, 1987.

Woodworth DA, et al: Bilateral congenital absence of maxillary lateral incisors. Am J Orthod Dentofacial Orthop 87:280–293, 1985.

Wyatt WE: Preventing adverse effects on the TMJ through orthodontic treatment. Am J Orthod Dentofacial Orthop 91:493–499, 1987.

Yamaguchi K, et al: A study of force application, amount of retarding force, and bracket width in sliding mechanics. Am J Orthod Dentofacial Orthop 109:50–56, 1996.

Young T, Smith R: Effects of orthodontics on the facial profile: a comparison of changes during nonextraction and four premolar extraction treatment. Am J Orthod Dentofacial Orthop 103:452–458, 1993.

Zachrisson BU: *Excellence in Orthodontics*. Syllabus.

Zachrisson BU: On excellence in finishing: Part 1. J Clin Orthod 7:460–482, 1986.

Index

Note: Page numbers in italics refer to illustrations; page numbers followed by t refer to tables.